The Lost Book of Medical Remedies

Discover The Healing Power of Herbal Remedies Inspired by Barbara O'Neill for Common Ailments to Naturally Improve your Wellness and Lifelong Health

By Barbara Parrish

Disclaimer

The information contained in this book is for general informational purposes only. The author makes no representations or warranties of any kind, express or implied, about the completeness, accuracy, reliability, suitability, or availability with respect to the contents of this book for any purpose. Any reliance you place on such information is therefore strictly at your own risk.

In no event will the author be liable for any loss or damage including without limitation, indirect or consequential loss or damage, or any loss or damage whatsoever arising from loss of data or profits arising out of or in connection with the use of this book. While every precaution has been taken in the preparation of this book, the author and publisher assume no responsibility for errors or omissions, or for damages resulting from the use of the information contained herein.

This book is not intended as a substitute for professional advice. Readers are advised to consult with qualified professionals for any questions or concerns they may have regarding their own situations. The views and opinions expressed in this book are those of the author and do not necessarily reflect the official policy or position of any other individual, agency, organization, employer, or company.

Contents

1

Getting Started with Herbs

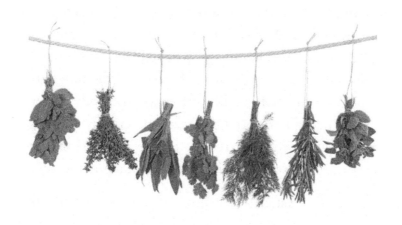

The world of medicinal plants is incredibly diverse, encompassing a vast array of species from every corner of the globe. From towering trees to delicate wildflowers, medicinal plants come in all shapes, sizes, and habitats, each with its own unique set of healing properties. Plants have been used as medicine by cultures around the world for thousands of years, providing relief from ailments ranging from the common cold to chronic diseases. Medicinal plants, whether grown in gardens, collected in the wild, or handed down through the years in traditional healing systems, provide a holistic approach to health and wellness that respects the body, mind, and spirit's interdependence.

At the heart of herbalism lies an understanding of the healing properties inherent in plants. From aromatic herbs that soothe the senses to potent botanicals with powerful medicinal effects, plants contain a wealth of bioactive compounds that contribute to their therapeutic value. Many medicinal plants are rich sources of vitamins, minerals, antioxidants, and other phytochemicals that support various aspects of health, including immune function, digestion, and circulation. Others possess specific pharmacological properties that make them effective remedies for specific ailments, such as anti-inflammatory, antimicrobial, and analgesic actions. By studying the unique chemical composition of plants and their interactions with the human body, herbalists can unlock the healing potential of nature's pharmacy, harnessing the power of plants to promote health and vitality.

Throughout history, diverse cultures have developed rich traditions of herbal medicine, passing down knowledge of medicinal plants from generation to generation. Traditional herbal systems such as Traditional Chinese Medicine (TCM), Ayurveda, and Western Herbalism offer valuable insights into the therapeutic properties of herbs and their applications for health and healing. In addition to traditional practices, modern herbalism incorporates scientific research and evidence-based practices to validate the efficacy and safety of herbal remedies. Advances in botany, phytochemistry, and pharmacology have shed light on the mechanisms of action behind herbal medicines, providing a deeper understanding of how plants exert their healing effects on the body. Today, herbal medicine continues to evolve, with herbalists and healthcare practitioners integrating traditional wisdom with contemporary knowledge to create effective and personalized treatment plans for individuals seeking natural alternatives to conventional medicine.

Herbalism is more than just a system of healing; it is a way of life that fosters a deep connection with the natural world. By working with medicinal plants, herbalists develop a profound appreciation for the cycles of nature, the wisdom of the earth, and the interconnectedness of all living beings. Through the act of growing, harvesting, and preparing herbs, herbalists cultivate a sense of reverence for the plants and the ecosystems that sustain them. They learn to listen to the subtle rhythms of nature, observing the changing seasons, the cycles of the moon, and the signs and signals of the plants themselves.

In turn, this connection with nature nourishes the body, mind, and spirit, promoting balance, vitality, and harmony within oneself and with the world around them. Herbalism becomes not only a means of healing but also a path to personal growth, self-discovery, and ecological stewardship.

Identifying and Harvesting Herbs Safely and Ethically

Identifying and harvesting herbs safely and ethically is essential for responsible herbalism and sustainable stewardship of our natural resources. In this section, we will explore the importance of proper plant identification, basic botanical terminology and characteristics, tips for ethical wildcrafting and foraging, and guidelines for sustainable harvesting practices. Proper plant identification is the cornerstone of safe and effective herbalism. With thousands of plant species in existence, many of which have similar appearances, it is crucial to accurately identify the plants you intend to use for medicinal purposes. Mistaken identity can lead to serious consequences, including poisoning or adverse reactions. To ensure accurate identification, herbalists must familiarize themselves with the botanical characteristics of each plant, including its leaves, flowers, stems, and roots. They should also consult reliable botanical references, field guides, and experienced mentors to confirm plant identities before harvesting or using them medicinally.

Basic Botanical Terminology and Characteristics

Understanding basic botanical terminology and characteristics is essential for accurate plant identification. Key terms include:

- Leaf Arrangement: How leaves are arranged on a stem (e.g., opposite, alternate, whorled).

- Leaf Shape: The overall shape of a leaf (e.g., ovate, lanceolate, palmate).

- Leaf Margin: The edge of a leaf (e.g., serrated, toothed, entire).

- Leaf Venation: The pattern of veins on a leaf (e.g., pinnate, palmate).

- Flower Structure: The arrangement and composition of flowers (e.g., solitary, inflorescence, umbel).

- Fruit Type: The structure that develops from the ovary of a flower (e.g., berry, capsule, nut).

By familiarizing themselves with these and other botanical characteristics, herbalists can confidently identify medicinal plants in their natural habitats.

Tips for Ethical Wildcrafting and Foraging

Wildcrafting and foraging for medicinal herbs can be a rewarding experience, but it is essential to do so responsibly and ethically. Here are some tips for ethical wildcrafting and foraging:

- Respect Nature: Harvest only what you need and leave enough plants behind to ensure their survival and reproduction.

- Know the Law: Familiarize yourself with local regulations and restrictions regarding wildcrafting and foraging, including permits and protected species.

- Harvest Mindfully: Choose harvesting sites carefully, avoiding areas with pollution, pesticide use, or other environmental hazards.

- Practice Leave-No-Trace: Minimize your impact on the environment by staying on designated trails, avoiding trampling sensitive habitats, and packing out any waste or litter.

- Give Thanks: Show gratitude to the plants, the land, and the ecosystems that sustain them by offering prayers, blessings, or offerings of gratitude.

Guidelines for Sustainable Harvesting Practices

Sustainable harvesting practices are essential for preserving wild plant populations and maintaining healthy ecosystems. Here are some guidelines for sustainable harvesting:

- Harvest Responsibly: Take only what you need and avoid overharvesting from wild populations.

- Promote Regeneration: Harvest from abundant species and encourage natural regeneration by leaving behind mature plants, seeds, and plant parts for propagation.

- Support Biodiversity: Avoid harvesting rare or endangered species and prioritize plants that are abundant and resilient.

- Rotate Harvesting Sites: Alternate harvesting locations to prevent depletion of plant populations in a single area.

- Monitor Impact: Regularly assess the health of harvested populations and adjust harvesting practices as needed to minimize negative impacts.

By following these guidelines, herbalists can ensure that their harvesting practices are sustainable, ethical, and respectful of the natural world.

Drying, Storing, and Preserving Herbs

Drying, storing, and preserving herbs are essential skills for any herbalist or home enthusiast seeking to extend the shelf life and potency of their botanical treasures. In this section, we will explore various methods for drying herbs, proper handling and storage techniques, tips for creating herbal infusions, blends, and mixtures, and creative ideas for herbal preservation.

Methods for Drying Herbs: Air Drying, Dehydrating, Oven Drying

1. Air Drying: Air drying is one of the oldest and simplest methods for preserving herbs. To air dry herbs, gather small bunches of freshly harvested herbs and tie them together with string or twine. Hang the bundles upside down in a warm, well-ventilated area away from direct sunlight. Allow the herbs to air dry until they are crisp and brittle, usually within 1 to 2 weeks depending on the humidity levels.

2. Dehydrating: Dehydrating herbs using a food dehydrator is a convenient and efficient way to preserve their potency. Simply spread freshly harvested herbs in a single layer on the dehydrator trays and set the temperature to the appropriate setting for herbs (usually around 95°F to 115°F or 35°C to 46°C). Allow the herbs to dehydrate until they are thoroughly dried, typically 4 to 12 hours depending on the moisture content and thickness of the herbs.

3. Oven Drying: Oven drying is another option for quickly drying herbs, especially when time is limited. To oven dry herbs, spread them in a single layer on a baking sheet lined with parchment paper. Place the baking sheet in a preheated oven set to the lowest temperature (usually around 140°F or 60°C) and leave the oven door slightly ajar to allow moisture to escape. Check the herbs frequently and remove them once they are completely dry.

Proper Handling and Storage Techniques to Preserve Herbal Potency

- Cooling and Cleaning: Allow freshly harvested herbs to cool completely before handling them, as heat can cause them to wilt and lose potency. Remove any damaged or discolored leaves and gently brush off any dirt or debris.

- Storage Containers: Store dried herbs in airtight containers such as glass jars, metal tins, or vacuum-sealed bags to protect them from moisture, light, and air. Label the containers with the name of the herb and the date of harvest to ensure freshness and potency.

- Storage Conditions: Store dried herbs in a cool, dark place away from direct sunlight, heat sources, and humidity. A pantry, cupboard, or drawer is ideal for preserving the flavor and potency of dried herbs.

Tips for Creating Herbal Infusions, Blends, and Mixtures

- Herbal Infusions: To make herbal infusions, steep dried herbs in hot water for several minutes to extract their medicinal properties and flavors. Strain the infusion and enjoy as a soothing tea or use it as a base for herbal remedies, culinary creations, and beauty products.

- Herbal Blends: Experiment with combining different dried herbs to create custom herbal blends tailored to your tastes and needs. Blend herbs for specific therapeutic purposes, culinary applications, or aromatic experiences.

- Herbal Mixtures: Mix dried herbs with other ingredients such as salts, sugars, oils, or vinegars to create flavorful and versatile herbal mixtures for cooking, seasoning, and preserving.

Creative Ideas for Herbal Preservation: Herbal Vinegars, Oils, and Butters

- Herbal Vinegars: Infuse dried herbs into vinegar to create herbal vinegars for culinary and medicinal use. Simply place dried herbs in a glass jar, cover them with vinegar, and let them steep for several weeks before straining and bottling the infused vinegar.

- Herbal Oils: Infuse dried herbs into oil to create herbal oils for cooking, massage, and skincare. Fill a glass jar with dried herbs and cover them with a carrier oil such as olive oil or jojoba oil. Let the mixture steep in a warm, sunny spot for several weeks before straining and storing the infused oil.

- Herbal Butters: Blend dried herbs into softened butter to create flavorful and aromatic herbal butters for spreading, cooking, and baking. Mix finely chopped dried herbs into softened butter and refrigerate until firm before using.

Tools and Equipment for Herbal Preparation

Having the right tools and equipment is essential for effectively preparing and utilizing medicinal herbs. In this section, we will explore essential tools for the herbal enthusiast, containers for herbal storage, equipment for herbal preparation, and advanced tools for herbalists.

Essential Tools for the Herbal Enthusiast

- Mortar and Pestle: A mortar and pestle is a classic tool for grinding herbs into powder or crushing them to release their aromatic oils. It allows for precise control over the texture and consistency of herbs and is essential for preparing herbal remedies, culinary creations, and aromatic blends.

- Herb Grinder: An herb grinder is a convenient tool for quickly and efficiently grinding larger quantities of herbs. It features sharp blades or teeth that shred herbs into fine particles, making them easier to work with in recipes, infusions, and tinctures.

- Kitchen Scale: A kitchen scale is indispensable for accurately measuring herbs and other ingredients in herbal preparations. It ensures consistency and precision in dosage and formulation, especially when working with potent herbs and medicinal compounds.

Containers for Herbal Storage

- Glass Jars: Glass jars are ideal for storing dried herbs, herbal infusions, tinctures, and oils. They provide airtight and light-resistant storage, preserving the potency and freshness of herbs for extended periods.

- Airtight Containers: Airtight containers, such as metal tins or plastic containers with tight-fitting lids, are suitable for storing dried herbs and herbal preparations. They protect herbs from exposure to air, moisture, and light, preventing degradation and loss of potency.

- Herbal Sachets: Herbal sachets are small pouches or bags filled with dried herbs and aromatic botanicals. They are used for scenting linens, drawers, and closets, as well as for making herbal bath blends and potpourri.

Equipment for Herbal Preparation

1. Strainers: Strainers are indispensable for separating liquid extracts from solid plant material in herbal infusions, decoctions, and tinctures. Choose strainers with fine mesh for removing small particles and debris from herbal preparations.

2. Cheesecloth: Cheesecloth is a versatile fabric that is commonly used in herbalism for straining and filtering herbal extracts, oils, and infusions. It allows for thorough filtration while allowing liquids to pass through easily.

3. Funnel: A funnel is a useful tool for transferring herbal preparations, oils, and tinctures into bottles and containers without spillage or waste. Look for funnels with a wide mouth and a narrow spout for easy pouring.

4. Dropper Bottles: Dropper bottles are essential for storing and dispensing liquid herbal extracts, tinctures, and essential oils. They feature a dropper cap or pipette for precise and controlled dosage, making them ideal for administering herbal remedies orally or topically.

Advanced Tools for Herbalists

1. Tincture Press: A tincture press is a specialized tool used for extracting the remaining liquid from herbal material after maceration or percolation. It ensures maximum yield and efficiency in tincture making, especially for large-scale herbal preparations.

2. Essential Oil Distiller: An essential oil distiller is a sophisticated apparatus used for steam distillation of aromatic plants to extract their essential oils. It allows herbalists to produce high-quality essential oils for aromatherapy, perfumery, and natural skincare.

3. Herbal Infusion Devices: Herbal infusion devices, such as herbal tea infusers and tea balls, are convenient tools for brewing loose herbs and botanicals into herbal teas and infusions. They allow for easy steeping and straining of herbs, resulting in flavorful and aromatic brews.

2

Herbal Pharmacology

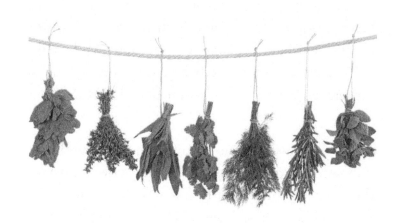

Barbara Parrish

Understanding Plant Chemistry

Understanding plant chemistry is akin to deciphering the language of nature's pharmaceutical laboratory. Plants, with their intricate biochemistry, have evolved an astonishing array of chemical compounds, often referred to as phytochemicals, which serve a multitude of functions, from defense against predators to attraction of pollinators. However, it is their medicinal properties that particularly captivate our attention. Among the diverse classes of phytochemicals, alkaloids, flavonoids, terpenes, and phenols stand out as key players in the pharmacological drama unfolding within the plant kingdom. Alkaloids, such as morphine and caffeine, possess potent physiological effects, ranging from pain relief to stimulation of the central nervous system. Flavonoids, abundant in fruits, vegetables, and medicinal herbs, exhibit antioxidant, anti-inflammatory, and immune-modulating properties, contributing to overall health and well-being.

Terpenes, with their characteristic aromatic profiles, offer a treasure trove of therapeutic potential. From the calming scent of lavender to the invigorating aroma of eucalyptus, terpenes influence our senses and physiology in profound ways, with antimicrobial, anti-inflammatory, and analgesic effects among their repertoire. Phenols, another class of phytochemicals, showcase antioxidant properties that protect against oxidative stress and inflammation, contributing to longevity and vitality. Delving into the intricacies of plant chemistry unveils a world of wonder and discovery for herbalists and researchers alike. By studying the chemical composition of plants and their interactions with biological systems, we gain insights into the mechanisms underlying their medicinal effects. Through meticulous analysis and experimentation, herbalists can identify the active constituents responsible for specific therapeutic actions and tailor herbal remedies to address individual health concerns.

Indeed, understanding plant chemistry is the key to unlocking the therapeutic potential of medicinal plants. It empowers us to harness the healing power of nature and formulate effective herbal remedies that promote health and vitality. As we delve deeper into the intricate web of phytochemical interactions, we gain a greater appreciation for the profound wisdom encoded within the botanical world, and the boundless potential it holds for human health and well-being.

Barbara Parrish

Key Active Compounds in Medicinal Plants

Medicinal plants are like treasure-pack of bioactive compounds, each with its own unique pharmacological prowess. Let's discuss some of the key players:

1. **Alkaloids** stand out with their nitrogen-rich structures, offering a myriad of physiological effects. Take morphine, for instance, derived from the opium poppy. It's renowned for its potent analgesic properties, offering relief from pain. Meanwhile, caffeine, a familiar companion in our morning cup of coffee, acts as a stimulant, boosting alertness and energy levels. Yet, alkaloids aren't limited to just these; they span a wide spectrum of functions, from sedative to stimulant, shaping the pharmacological landscape of medicinal plants.

2. **Flavonoids** bring their polyphenolic prowess to the table, packing a punch with antioxidant, anti-inflammatory, and immune-boosting abilities. Found abundantly in fruits, vegetables, and medicinal herbs like chamomile and ginkgo, they act as natural defenders, shielding the body from oxidative stress and inflammation. With their vibrant hues and potent properties, flavonoids are not just mere pigments; they are nature's remedy for bolstering health and vitality.

3. **Terpenes**, aromatic compounds with a diverse array of biological activities, infuse medicinal plants with their distinct fragrances and potent effects. From the soothing scent of lavender to the refreshing aroma of peppermint and eucalyptus, terpenes offer more than just olfactory delight; they deliver antimicrobial, anti-inflammatory, and analgesic relief, making them indispensable in essential oils and herbal remedies alike.

4. **Phenols** emerge as antioxidants, combating oxidative stress and inflammation with their protective powers. Herbs like rosemary, thyme, and sage are rich in these compounds, offering not just culinary flair but also medicinal benefits. Phenolic compounds serve as guardians of health, fortifying the body against the ravages of free radicals and inflammatory processes.

5. **Glycosides** add a sweet touch to medicinal plants, binding sugars to their medicinal compounds. Cardiac glycosides found in foxglove and anthraquinone glycosides in senna illustrate the diverse pharmacological potential of these compounds. Whether regulating heart function or aiding in bowel movements, glycosides play a vital role in the medicinal arsenal of plants.

Understanding the pharmacological intricacies of these bioactive compounds is akin to unlocking nature's pharmacy. With each compound offering a unique set of benefits, herbalists and researchers alike can harness the power of medicinal plants to formulate effective remedies tailored to individual needs.

Methods of Herbal Preparation

Herbalists, with their deep understanding of plant medicine, wield an array of methods to prepare medicinal concoctions that harness the healing power of nature. Here's an exploration of some common methods:

1. Infusions gently coax out the soluble constituents of dried herbs by steeping them in hot water. This method is perfect for delicate plant parts like leaves and flowers, allowing volatile oils, flavonoids, and vitamins to gracefully infuse into the water. Herbal teas, with their comforting warmth and therapeutic properties, are the quintessential example of infusions, offering a soothing sip of wellness.

2. Decoctions, akin to infusions but with a bolder approach, call for a hearty boil of tougher plant components such as roots, bark, and seeds. By subjecting these robust parts to the vigorous embrace of boiling water, both soluble and insoluble constituents are coaxed out, resulting in a brew that packs a potent punch. Decoctions, with their robust flavors and concentrated medicinal benefits, are often favored when a stronger dose is needed to tackle ailments.

3. Tinctures epitomize the essence of concentration, capturing the essence of herbs in a potent liquid form. Through maceration or percolation, plant material surrenders its treasures to alcohol or another solvent, resulting in a concentrated elixir that boasts both efficacy and longevity. Tinctures, with their convenience and shelf stability, stand as stalwart allies in the quest for herbal healing, offering a convenient and potent dosage of plant medicine.

4. Powders offer a versatile canvas for herbalists to work their magic, transforming dried herbs into a finely ground form that can be easily encapsulated or incorporated into various preparations. With the aid of mortar and pestle or herb grinder, plant material is pulverized into a fine dust, ready to be deployed in herbal teas, infusions, or even culinary creations. Herbal powders, with their adaptability and ease of use, serve as the foundation for a myriad of herbal remedies.

5. Oils and Salves bring herbal medicine to the realm of skincare and topical applications, infusing carrier oils or beeswax with the essence of dried herbs. Through gentle heating or steeping, the medicinal properties of herbs permeate the oil or wax, creating a soothing balm or salve that nourishes the skin and soothes ailments. Whether massaging away muscle tension or nourishing dry skin, herbal oils and salves offer a luxurious and effective way to experience the healing touch of plants.

Dosage and Administration Guidelines

Getting the right amount and using herbs properly is super important to make sure they work well and don't cause harm. How much herb to take depends on lots of things, like how strong the herbs are, what you're using them for, and stuff about you, like your age, weight, and health. Herbal experts and doctors use science and old knowledge to figure out the right amount of herbs for different situations. They might change the dose depending on how you react and if you're taking other meds, to make sure everything goes smoothly.

You can take herbs in different ways: swallowing them, putting them on your skin, breathing them in, or using them outside on your body. Each way has its own perks, depending on what you need and where you need it to work.

By sticking to the right dose and way of using herbs, experts and folks can get the most good out of them without worrying too much about bad stuff happening.

3

Key Medicinal Plants

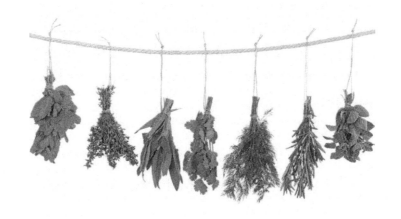

Barbara Parrish

Agrimony, Agrimonia eupatoria

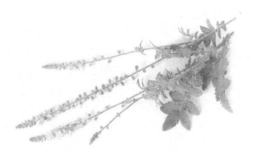

Composition:

- **Primary Components:** Contains tannins, which are responsible for its potent astringent properties; flavonoids, which provide antioxidant benefits; and volatile oils.
- **Other Phytochemicals:** Also includes catechins and quercetin, which contribute to its health benefits.

Agrimony, also known as sticklewort, cocklebur, or church steeples, hails from Europe and has since spread throughout North America. This charming plant boasts spiky clusters of petite yellow blossoms and belongs to the Rosaceae, or Rose, family. Sporting a rich green hue, this perennial plant features a coarse stem blanketed in fine hairs that aid in seed dispersal. It stands about two feet tall, with serrated, feather-like leaves that are larger at the bottom (around 7 inches) and gradually reduce in size towards the top of the stem. Its roots are sturdy, deep-set rhizomes. The plant produces short-stemmed flowers with a delightful apricot scent, blooming from June through September on elongated terminal spikes. Each bloom resembles a cup adorned with rows of hook-shaped bristles at the rim. The flowers consist of five sepals and five rounded, yellow petals, each encircled by 5 to 20 stamens. The fruit features cockleburs, or hooked bristles, that latch onto animals, thereby dispersing the seeds.

Uses:

1. Brew the leaves for a soothing tea, or toss fresh flowers into homemade beer or wine for an extra kick of flavor.

2. Slipping a few leaves beneath your pillow at bedtime could help you drift off to sleep.

3. Agrimony is a boon for wound care, halting heavy bleeding and encouraging clot formation, thanks to its tannin content and astringent nature. It also possesses antibacterial and anti-inflammatory qualities. You can either use Agrimony tea as a cleansing wash for wounds and various skin conditions or mash up fresh leaves to create a healing poultice.

4. Sipping on Agrimony Tea may settle digestive troubles, acting as a restorative tonic for the gut.

5. For a gentle eye rinse, blend Agrimony Tea with an equal measure of boiled water that's been allowed to cool.

6. A head wrap made from fresh agrimony leaves could be your ally against migraines; it might even help you enjoy a deep, restful sleep if you wear it overnight.

Preparation:

1. Tea (Infusion):

- To make agrimony tea, steep 1-2 teaspoons of dried agrimony herb in boiling water for about 10-15 minutes. This helps to extract the tannins and other beneficial compounds.
- Consumption Advice: The tea can be consumed two to three times a day, especially to harness its astringent properties for throat and mouth health.

2. Tincture

- Agrimony can also be used to make a tincture by soaking the herb in alcohol (such as vodka) for a few weeks. This method extracts a broader range of soluble compounds.
- Usage: Typically, tinctures are used in small doses (a few drops), and can be added to water or tea before consumption.

3. Topical Application:

- Poultice: For skin irritations or mild inflammatory skin conditions, a poultice made from fresh or dried agrimony can be applied directly to the skin. This involves macerating the plant material to form a paste and applying it to the affected area.

Safety and Considerations:

Interactions: Due to its astringent properties, agrimony may interfere with the absorption of certain medications. It's important to consult a healthcare provider if you are on medication, particularly those for digestion or related to mineral absorption.

Pregnancy and Breastfeeding: There is insufficient research on the effects of agrimony during pregnancy and breastfeeding, so it is best avoided during these times.
Allergies: As with many herbs, some people may experience allergic reactions to agrimony. It's a good practice to test a small amount on your skin before using it more broadly, especially if applied topically.

Horse Chestnut, Aesculus hippocastanum

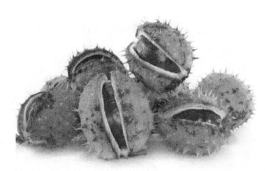

Composition:

- **Active Ingredients:** Contains a compound called aescin, which is thought to strengthen vein walls and reduce inflammation.
- **Other Components:** Also includes flavonoids, coumarins (including aesculin), and tannins.

Horse chestnut seeds, those glossy brown "conkers" British kids gather in the fall, are proven to ease varicose vein symptoms and aid in their healing. Whether you swallow it or use it as a cream, horse chestnut can firm up your body's tissues and lessen the discomfort and swelling associated with varicose veins. It's also great for cutting down on fluid buildup. Originating from the mountainous forests stretching from the Balkans to the Himalayas, horse chestnut is now grown for its beauty and shade across the globe, particularly in Europe. You can grow it from seeds in either fall or spring, and collect its leaves in summer and bark and seeds in fall.

Uses:

1. Loads of studies back up the medicinal benefits of horse chestnut for vein-related issues like varicose veins, venous ulcers, hemorrhoids, and even frostbite. A study out of London in 1996 showed that horse chestnut extract can match compression stockings in treating varicose veins. In Germany, it's common practice to use horse chestnut extracts and aescin for these vein issues.

2. A 2006 review by the Cochrane Database looked at horse chestnut extract for chronic venous insufficiency, which includes symptoms like leg swelling and various vein problems. They found that horse chestnut extract is safe and effective for short-term treatment of this condition.

3. While horse chestnut can be good for the heart and arteries, it really shines when it comes to treating veins. It strengthens vein walls, preventing issues like varicose veins and hemorrhoids. It also tackles edema by stopping fluid from leaking out of veins and helps fluid return to the circulatory system. People take horse chestnut internally for leg ulcers, varicose veins, and frostbite, and apply it directly to the skin as a lotion, gel, or ointment. A bark or leaf brew can be used as a skin-tightening lotion for varicose veins.

4. Over in France, they've used an oil made from the seeds to rub on rheumatism.

5. Horse chestnut is also used as a chest remedy. In Turkey, it's been used for treating horses' chest conditions, and in the U.S., a leaf concoction has been handy for whooping cough.

Preparation:

1. **Seed Extract:** This is the most common medicinal form. Commercial preparations of horse chestnut seed extract (often abbreviated as HCSE) are standardized to contain 16 to 20% aescin. These extracts are typically made using a process that eliminates the toxic aesculin component.

2. **Tincture:**

- Grind the horse chestnut seeds to a fine powder (note: commercially available products undergo processes to remove toxicity).
- Place the ground seeds in a jar and cover with a high-proof alcohol, such as vodka, to draw out the soluble active ingredients.
- Seal the jar and store it in a dark, cool place for about 4 to 6 weeks, shaking it daily.
- After the maceration period, strain the mixture through a cheesecloth or fine mesh, bottle the liquid, and label it clearly.
- Note: Homemade preparations might not effectively remove toxic compounds and are generally not recommended.

Safety and Considerations:

1. Do not attempt to make homemade horse chestnut preparations that require consumption or topical application on broken skin without ensuring that all toxic components are removed.

2. Always consult with a healthcare provider before using horse chestnut, especially if you are pregnant, nursing, or taking medication for diabetes or blood thinning.

Anise Hyssop, Agastache foeniculum

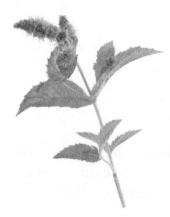

Composition:

• **Primary Components:** Contains essential oils, including anethole, which gives it its distinctive licorice flavor, as well as flavonoids, tannins, and other phytochemicals.
• **Other Nutrients:** Rich in vitamins and minerals, including vitamin C, calcium, and magnesium.

Anise hyssop, which is also known by names like blue giant hyssop, lavender giant hyssop, elk mint, and licorice mint, is part of the mint family, Lamiaceae. This plant is originally from the northern and central regions of North America. Standing between 2 and 5 feet tall, it features vibrant green, slightly jagged leaves with a soft, white fuzz on the bottom. When the plant sprouts new leaves, they often have a purplish hue. Anise hyssop smells a bit like a mix between mint and anise, and it has a somewhat woody nature with stems that are typically bare of hair. Its roots spread out in a branching fashion. From July to September, the plant blossoms with small, lilac-blue flowers in clustered spikes.

Uses:

1. Anise hyssop is great for sweetening dishes or brewing tea, and you can enjoy its leaves and flowers fresh, cooked, or dried for flavoring.

2. If you're dealing with skin infections, cuts, or burns, try a poultice made from anise hyssop leaves. Either moisten dried leaves or mash up fresh ones, apply them to the troubled spot, and cover with a clean cloth. These leaves are known for their anti-bacterial and anti-viral traits.

3. Sipping anise hyssop tea with your meals can help make digestion smoother and keep bloating and gas at bay.

4. If diarrhea's giving you trouble, anise hyssop tea might be your friend. Keep drinking it throughout the day, even after things settle, to keep the problem from coming back.

5. For those pesky colds, the flu, or chest congestion, anise hyssop tea can help clear out that mucus.

6. You can also use anise hyssop essential oil on your skin as an antiviral remedy for Herpes Simplex I and II, and drinking the tea can fight the virus from within.

7. If poison ivy's got you itching, washing with anise hyssop infusion might just soothe your skin.

8. Battling athlete's foot, fungal skin infections, or yeast issues? Soak the affected area in a strong anise hyssop infusion bath. Do this daily until you see the infection clear up.

Preparation:

1. Tea (Infusion):

- Steep 1-2 teaspoons of dried anise hyssop leaves in hot water for about 5-10 minutes. This extracts the flavorful compounds and medicinal properties.
- Flavor Enhancements: Anise hyssop tea can be enjoyed on its own or combined with other herbs like mint or lemon balm for added flavor complexity.

Safety and Considerations:

Allergic Reactions: Some individuals may be allergic to plants in the mint family, to which anise hyssop belongs. If you have allergies to plants like mint, basil, or oregano, use anise hyssop with caution.

Pregnancy and Breastfeeding: Limited information is available on the safety of anise hyssop during pregnancy and breastfeeding, so it's best to avoid large amounts.

Medication Interactions: Anise hyssop may interact with certain medications, particularly those metabolized by the liver. If you are taking medications, consult with a healthcare professional before using anise hyssop medicinally.

Garlic Allium sativum

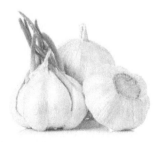

Composition:
- Primary Components: Contains allicin, which is responsible for its distinctive smell and many of its therapeutic effects. When garlic cloves are crushed, chopped, or chewed, this compound is formed from the precursor compound alliin.
- Other Phytochemicals: Includes sulfides, saponins, phenols, and flavonoids.

Garlic, with its strong smell and flavor, is an excellent natural remedy that's completely safe for use at home and packs a punch against numerous health issues. It fights off various infections, particularly in the respiratory system, and is beneficial for lowering cholesterol, aiding blood flow issues like hypertension, and managing blood sugar, which is particularly helpful for those with type 2 diabetes. Originating from central Asia, garlic is now cultivated all over the globe. It's grown from the segments of the bulb and harvested in the late summer of the following year.

Uses:

1. Over a thousand studies have highlighted garlic's medicinal benefits. These include its ability to reduce high levels of blood fats, including cholesterol, prevent blood clots, lower high blood pressure, decrease elevated blood sugar, and fight infections.

2. Garlic has long been revered for its curative properties. Before modern antibiotics came into play, it was a go-to remedy for a wide range of infections, such as tuberculosis and typhoid. During World War I, it was even used to treat wounds.

3. Garlic is a top choice for fighting chest infections. It's effective against colds, the flu, and ear infections, and it can also help clear out mucus.

4. If you're dealing with digestive infections, garlic can be quite beneficial. It also eliminates intestinal parasites.

5. To prevent circulatory issues and strokes, garlic is a star. It keeps your blood flowing smoothly, cuts down cholesterol, and helps with blood pressure control.

6. Garlic's healing scope is broad, tackling everything from hay fever and asthma to an enlarged prostate and osteoarthritis. It's also handy when paired with conventional antibiotics to minimize side effects like diarrhea. With strong antifungal properties, it's effective for fungal skin conditions, whether taken orally or applied topically. Plus, it's recognized for its anti-cancer properties, particularly in safeguarding against stomach and colon cancers.

Preparation

1. Raw Use:

- Simply peel the garlic clove, mince, slice, or crush it to add to dishes. The method of preparation affects the intensity and sharpness of the flavor; crushing produces a stronger flavor than slicing.

2. Cooked Use:

- Garlic can be roasted whole in the oven, which mellows its pungency and brings out its natural sweetness. To roast garlic, slice off the top of the head of garlic to expose the cloves, drizzle with olive oil, wrap in foil, and bake at 400°F (about 204°C) for 30-35 minutes.
- Sautéed or stir-fried garlic can be added to recipes for a less intense but flavorful addition.

3. Medicinal Preparations:

- Garlic Oil: Peel and mince several cloves of garlic, and then simmer them gently in olive oil over very low heat for about 20 minutes. Strain the oil and store in a sealed container in the refrigerator. This oil can be used for culinary purposes or as a topical remedy for conditions like ear infections.
- Garlic Tea: A less common preparation, involving steeping minced garlic in hot water for several minutes. This can be drunk (often with honey to soften the taste) for relief from cold or flu symptoms.

Safety and Considerations:

Consumption Considerations: Eating garlic in food is generally safe for most people. However, consuming large amounts of raw garlic, especially on an empty stomach, can cause gastrointestinal irritation or discomfort.

Allergies and Medication Interactions: People taking blood thinners should use garlic cautiously due to its potential to amplify the effects of these medications. Always consult with a healthcare provider if you're considering taking garlic as a supplement or if you have a condition that might be affected by increased garlic intake.

Remember, if you're thinking of giving garlic to kids under 12 as a medicine, or if you're on blood-thinning medication, it's best to get advice from a healthcare professional first.

Ashwagandha, Withania somnifera

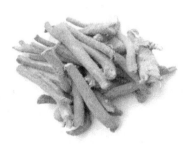

Composition:
- Primary Components: Contains withanolides, which are steroidal lactones that contribute to its therapeutic effects, including its adaptogenic and anti-inflammatory properties.
- Other Phytochemicals: Alkaloids (like withanine), saponins, and iron.

Ashwagandha, also known as Withania somnifera, belongs to the Solanaceae or nightshade family. It's commonly referred to as Winter Cherry or Indian Ginseng because of its significant role in traditional Ayurvedic healing practices. Renowned for its adaptogenic properties, Ashwagandha is prized for its ability to rejuvenate and provide relief from various health issues. This herb is indigenous to India but has adapted well to herb gardens across the U.S., thriving as a perennial in regions free from frost. It favors sandy or rocky soils, enjoys both full and partial sunshine, and prefers conditions that are somewhat arid.

Uses:

1. While the plant itself isn't typically consumed, its seeds are handy in making plant-based cheeses. Plus, its leaves can be brewed into a soothing Ashwagandha Tea.

2. Ashwagandha is a supporter of adrenal health and is known to help with what's often called "adrenal fatigue." However, a more precise term for this condition is hypothalamic-pituitary-adrenal (HPA) axis dysfunction, which is essentially our body's stress management system. Ashwagandha works to harmonize this system.

3. It's been a go-to remedy for easing anxiety, boosting mental clarity, enhancing vitality, and lifting overall life quality. Ashwagandha also acts as a mood stabilizer and can alleviate depression symptoms, offering benefits similar to those of anti-anxiety and anti-depressant medications but without the unwanted side effects like drowsiness or insomnia.

4. Ashwagandha has been shown to significantly lower cortisol, a stress hormone that plays a role in blood sugar regulation and abdominal fat storage, especially in those dealing with chronic stress.

5. For individuals with diabetes, Ashwagandha is a boon, as it can help in lowering blood sugar levels, potentially improving insulin sensitivity, and reducing inflammation.

6. The herb demonstrates anti-cancer properties, inhibiting the growth of tumors and destroying cancer cells. It's particularly helpful in managing breast, lung, stomach, ovarian, and colon cancers due to its antioxidant capabilities and immune system support. Beyond slowing cancer cell growth, it assists the body in coping with the adverse effects of traditional cancer treatments by boosting immunity and life quality. It also promotes white blood cell production, aiding infection resistance in cancer patients.

7. Those who incorporate Ashwagandha into their regimen for at least eight weeks often report enhanced joint function and a decrease in joint pain, particularly related to rheumatoid arthritis.

8. Ashwagandha plays a role in modulating immune responses by dialing down stress hormones, curbing inflammation, boosting white blood cell counts, and ramping up immunoglobulin production.

9. When it comes to sexual health, Ashwagandha is a natural enhancer. It can increase testosterone levels and male fertility. After using it for around three months, men may notice a rise in sperm count, volume, and motility. For women, it can heighten arousal, improve lubrication, and intensify orgasms.

Preparation:

1. Powder from Dried Roots:

- Preparation: The roots are cleaned, dried, and ground into a fine powder. This powder can be used in various ways, including capsules, teas, or mixed into foods or smoothies.
- Typically, it's recommended to take about 3 to 6 grams of the powdered root daily, though starting doses might be lower to gauge tolerance.

2. Ashwagandha Tea:

- Simple Tea Preparation: Boil a teaspoon of ashwagandha powder in water for 10 minutes. Strain and drink. This can be sweetened with honey or mixed with other herbal teas to improve taste.
- Nighttime Beverage: A popular way to consume ashwagandha is to mix the powder into warm milk with honey before bedtime, enhancing its stress-reducing and sleep-promoting effects.

3. Tincture:

- Alcohol Extraction: An ashwagandha tincture involves soaking the dried root in alcohol to extract the active compounds. This is taken in small quantities, usually measured in drops.
- Usage: Typically, tinctures are more concentrated than powders, so the dosage might be several drops up to three times a day.

Safety and Considerations:

Pregnancy and Breastfeeding: Ashwagandha is not recommended for pregnant or breastfeeding women due to potential effects on hormonal balance.

Thyroid Conditions: Because it can potentiate thyroid hormone production, those with thyroid disorders should consult a healthcare provider before starting ashwagandha.

Autoimmune Diseases: People with autoimmune conditions such as rheumatoid arthritis, lupus, or Hashimoto's thyroiditis should use ashwagandha with caution as it might stimulate the immune system.

Medication Interactions: Ashwagandha may interact with medications for diabetes, hypertension, and sedatives due to its effects on blood sugar and blood pressure, as well as its sedative properties.

Aloe Vera, Aloes

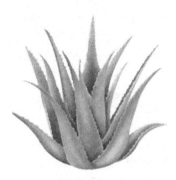

Composition:
- **Primary Components:** The aloe vera leaf contains a clear gel made up of water, 20 minerals, 12 vitamins, 18 amino acids, and 200 active plant compounds (phytonutrients), including enzymes, triterpenes, glycoproteins, sterols, lignin, and salicylic acids.
- The yellow sap called latex, found just under the skin of the leaf, contains compounds known as anthraquinones, including aloin, which have potent laxative properties.

Aloe vera, a plant native to Africa, is often grown in homes as a decorative plant, and it boasts two main therapeutic applications. The transparent gel found in its leaves is an excellent remedy for healing cuts and burns quickly, while also preventing infections. The dried yellow sap, called "bitter aloes," acts as a potent laxative, ideal for relieving temporary constipation. Originating from eastern and southern Africa, aloe vera thrives in tropical climates and is widely cultivated around the globe. (Note that aloe vera plants kept in pots tend to have less anthraquinone content.) You can propagate aloe vera by separating small, rooted offshoots. To harvest the gel and bitter liquid, simply slice the leaves and let them drain.

Uses:

1. Studies from the 1930s onward in the U.S. and Russia have revealed that the clear gel can significantly heal wounds, ulcers, and burns by forming a protective layer and accelerating the healing process, partly thanks to aloectin B, which boosts the immune system.

2. Aloe vera has been celebrated as a beauty aid for centuries—legend has it that Cleopatra swore by it for her stunning looks.

3. In the 1950s, the West caught on to aloe vera's benefits, especially for treating burns, including those caused by radiation.

4. Aloe vera makes for an outstanding immediate treatment for burns, cuts, scalds, and sunburns. Snapping off a leaf releases the calming gel, which can be directly applied to the injured area.

5. The gel is also beneficial for various skin issues that require soothing and tightening, and it may even help with varicose veins to some extent.

6. Aloe vera's protective and healing powers also extend internally; the gel can be consumed to aid with conditions like peptic ulcers and irritable bowel syndrome.

7. The bitter yellow liquid in the leaves contains anthraquinones, which are strong laxatives. They trigger contractions in the colon, usually leading to a bowel movement within 8 to 12 hours after intake. In small amounts, the herb's bitter qualities can kick-start digestion, while larger doses act as laxatives and purgatives.

Preparation:

1. Extracting Aloe Vera Gel:

- Harvesting: Select mature leaves from the bottom of the plant, as they contain a higher concentration of active ingredients.
- Peeling: Cut off the serrated edges of the leaf. Carefully peel the outer layer of the leaf with a knife, exposing the clear inner gel.
- Extracting: Scoop out the gel using a spoon or slice the leaf into sections and press out the gel. It's important to avoid the yellow aloe latex if you're using the gel for topical application, as it can be irritating to the skin.

2. Storing Aloe Vera Gel:

- Short Term: The fresh gel can be stored in the refrigerator for about a week in an airtight container.
- Long Term: For longer storage, aloe gel can be frozen in ice cube trays and then transferred to freezer bags, where it can be stored for several months.

Safety and Considerations:

Topical Use: Generally safe, but some individuals may experience allergic reactions. It's a good practice to perform a patch test on a small area of skin before widespread use.

Oral Consumption: The aloe latex contains aloin, which can be harsh on the gastrointestinal system, causing diarrhea and cramps. Products made for consumption should be purified to remove aloin (often labeled as "decolorized"). Always consult a healthcare provider before starting any new dietary supplement, especially if you have pre-existing conditions or are pregnant.

Black-Eyed Susan, Rudbeckia hirta

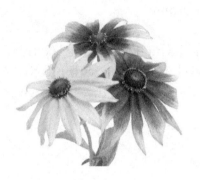

Composition:

• **Primary Components:** Contains various compounds including flavonoids, which are known for their antioxidant properties, and essential oils.
• **Parts Used:** Traditionally, the roots, leaves, and flowers have been used in various preparations.

Black-eyed Susan, part of the Aster/Sunflower family, thrives across the eastern and central regions of North America. Known by various names such as brown-eyed Susan, hairy coneflower, and gloriosa daisy, among others, this plant loves basking in the sun and grows best in soil that's either moist or somewhat dry.

Typically an annual, though occasionally a perennial, Black-eyed Susan can reach heights of 3 feet and spread out to about 1.5 feet. Its leaves, which are about 4 to 7 inches long, are rough to the touch due to coarse hairs. The plant sprouts branched stems from a single taproot, and it reproduces solely by seeds. Keep an eye out for its blooms in the late summer and early fall; they feature a dark brown or black center surrounded by vibrant yellow petals and measure roughly 4 inches across.

Uses:

1. Black-eyed Susan has been traditionally harnessed to combat colds, flu, infections, inflammation, and even snake bites. The roots, and occasionally the leaves, are favored for their immune-boosting and infection-fighting properties.

2. Drinking a root infusion is a common remedy for colds and flu—just keep sipping it daily until you're feeling back to normal.

3. The Chippewa have historically brewed Black-eyed Susan Root Tea to address worms in children.

4. For snake bites, a poultice made from the crushed leaves or ground root can help. Apply it to the bite, wrap it up, and leave it on to reduce swelling.

5. Soothing irritated skin is another benefit. Warm root infusions can gently cleanse sores, cuts, scrapes, and swollen areas.

6. Got an earache? Fresh root sap or juice can work wonders. A couple of drops in the ear twice a day should do the trick until the infection subsides.

7. Similar to Echinacea, the roots can stimulate the immune system, making it a go-to for fighting off minor illnesses. However, those with autoimmune conditions should proceed with caution due to its stimulating effects.

8. Lastly, Black-eyed Susan is known to have compounds that can take on the bacteria responsible for tuberculosis.

Preparation:

1. Tea Preparation:

- Leaves and Flowers: These can be dried and used to make an herbal tea. Simply steep 1-2 teaspoons of dried leaves or flowers in hot water for about 10 minutes.
- Roots: The roots can also be dried and chopped into small pieces, then used to make a decoction. This involves boiling the roots in water for about 20 minutes to extract their active compounds.

2. Tincture:

- A tincture can be made from the fresh or dried flowers and leaves. Soak the plant material in a mixture of water and alcohol (typically vodka or grain alcohol) for several weeks, shaking periodically. Strain and store in a dark bottle for use.

3. Poultice:

- Fresh leaves and flowers can be crushed or mashed into a poultice and applied topically to wounds, burns, or skin infections. This method utilizes the soothing properties of the plant to aid in healing.

Safety and Considerations:

Allergic Reactions: As with many plants, it is possible to have an allergic reaction. It's recommended to do a patch test by applying a small amount of any new herbal preparation to the skin in a less sensitive area before using it more broadly.

Pregnancy and Breastfeeding: There is insufficient research on the effects of Black-Eyed Susan during pregnancy and breastfeeding, so it is best to avoid use during these times unless directed by a healthcare provider.

Medical Conditions and Medications: If you are on medication or have a health condition, consult with a healthcare provider before using herbal remedies, including those made from Black-Eyed Susan, to avoid potential interactions or side effects.

Galangal, Alpinia officinarum

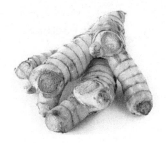

Composition:

• Primary Components: Contains volatile oils, including galangin, gingerol, and galanolactone, which contribute to its distinctive sharp, spicy flavor and health benefits.
• Other Phytochemicals: Also includes flavonoids, terpenes, and phenolic acids.

Similar to its ginger family relatives, galangal offers a cozy and soothing effect on our digestive system. It's known for its delightfully fragrant and slightly spicy flavor, making it a go-to for when you need to bring a little extra heat to your body's core. Europe got its first taste of galangal around the 9th century, and the German mystic Hildegard of Bingen praised it as a divine gift to keep sickness at bay, calling it the "spice of life." This plant hails from the grassy lands of southern China and the broader Southeast Asian region. These days, galangal is grown across tropical Asia, both for its culinary zest and medicinal benefits. Come spring, growers split and replant its rhizomes, which thrive in well-drained soil with a bit of shade. After 4 to 6 years, the mature rhizomes are gathered at the season's close and can be used either fresh or dried.

Uses

1. It's been found to pack an antibacterial punch, particularly against the Staphylococcus aureus bacteria, a common culprit in ear, nose, and throat infections.

2. Lab studies have shown that galangal is pretty effective at taking on fungi, including the notorious Candida albicans.

3. Back in 2001, a study revealed that a potent mix of ginger and galangal extracts helped ease knee osteoarthritis symptoms.

4. Over in India and southwestern Asia, folks turn to galangal as a remedy for stomach issues, inflammation, coughs, and in traditional Chinese medicine, it's used to combat abdominal pain, vomiting, hiccups, and even cold-induced diarrhea.

5. Arabian physicians introduced galangal to Europe over a millennium ago. It's commonly used in Western remedies for gas, indigestion, vomiting, and stomachaches. A brewed concoction can even help with mouth ulcers and tender gums. Plus, it's been a go-to for preventing seasickness, which makes sense given its motion sickness-fighting reputation.

6. When dealing with intestinal candidiasis, galangal can be part of a herbal anti-fungal team to tackle the condition.

Preparation:

1. Fresh Galangal:

- Preparation for Cooking: Fresh galangal root can be prepared by washing it thoroughly and slicing or mincing it. The skin is typically tough, so it's often removed before using. Fresh galangal can be grated or ground with a mortar and pestle to release its flavors.
- Storage: Fresh galangal can be wrapped in a damp cloth or paper towel, placed in a plastic bag, and stored in the refrigerator for up to three weeks. To extend its shelf life, it can also be frozen.

2. Dried Galangal:

- Rehydration: Dried galangal needs to be rehydrated before use. Soak it in hot water for about 30 minutes, or until it softens.
- Ground Galangal: Dried and ground galangal is available and can be used directly in recipes, although its flavor is less potent than fresh.

3. Galangal Powder:

- Direct Use: Galangal powder can be used as a spice in cooking and as a supplement in teas or smoothies.

Safety and Considerations:

General Tolerance: Galangal is generally considered safe when used as a food ingredient. The amounts typically used in cooking are unlikely to cause adverse effects.

Medicinal Use Precautions: When used medicinally in larger quantities, it's best to consult with a healthcare provider, especially for those who are pregnant, breastfeeding, or have existing health conditions.

Interaction with Medications: Like ginger, galangal may interact with medications, especially those that affect blood clotting, such as anticoagulants.

Boneset, Eupatorium perfoliatum

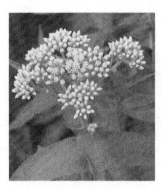

Composition:

• **Primary Components:** Contains sesquiterpene lactones, flavonoids, and pyrrolizidine alkaloids, which contribute to its medicinal effects. The presence of these alkaloids also necessitates caution due to their potential toxicity.

• **Parts Used:** The leaves and flowering tops are the parts most commonly used for medicinal purposes.

Boneset, an herb named for its historical use in alleviating dengue fever, often referred to as break-bone fever, is a go-to remedy for fevers and respiratory illnesses like colds and influenza. This perennial plant is indigenous to North America and belongs to the Aster/Sunflower family. It's also called feverwort. With its tall, fuzzy stems that can reach heights between 2 and 4 feet and branch out at the top, boneset is easily recognizable. Its large, paired leaves join at the base, are lance-shaped with fine teeth and distinct veins, and measure 4 to 8 inches in length, with the lower leaves being larger. The leaf surface is coarse, while the underside is softer, sticky, and speckled. The leaves are unique because they appear to be pierced by the stem or are united at their base. Boneset blooms from July to September, presenting numerous flower heads with 10 to 20 white florets, each surrounded by a single row of bristly hairs. The plant emits a mildly aromatic scent and has a taste that is both astringent and intensely bitter. While the plant's size and other characteristics can vary widely, these are some of its distinguishing features.

Uses

1. The flowers and leaves of boneset are the parts utilized for medicinal purposes. It's safer to use them dried since fresh boneset can be somewhat toxic. The herb is known for its diverse medicinal uses, including acting as an antispasmodic, inducing sweat, stimulating bile production, serving as an emetic, reducing fever, functioning as a laxative and purgative, providing stimulation, and expanding blood vessels.

2. When it comes to combating common colds, flus, and respiratory infections, boneset is an excellent option. It hampers mucus production, breaks down phlegm, and aids in its expulsion from the body. It also combats viral and bacterial infections and encourages sweating to help bring down fevers. Starting boneset treatment early in an illness can lead to milder symptoms and a quicker recovery. A tincture is the simplest form to administer.

3. Although dengue fever, which thrives in tropical climates, hasn't become widespread in the United States yet, it's likely only a matter of time before we see it here. Boneset is the herb of choice to fight off dengue, a painful mosquito-transmitted disease that causes high fevers and intense muscle and bone pain. It helps lower fevers and address the root causes of the disease, providing relief from the intense pain.

4. Traditional uses of boneset by Native Americans include the treatment of malaria. It promotes sweating, which in turn helps to reduce the fevers associated with malaria and diminishes the disease's severity.

5. While boneset is also used to treat yellow fever and typhoid, it's not as potent for these conditions as it is for dengue fever and malaria. Its primary benefit in these cases is its fever-reducing ability.

Preparation:

1. Tea (Infusion):

- Simple Preparation: Steep 1-2 teaspoons of dried boneset leaves and flowers in a cup of boiling water for about 10 to 15 minutes. Strain the leaves and flowers out before drinking.
- Dosage: Typically, the tea is consumed hot and can be taken several times a day, especially to treat fever and flu symptoms. It is recommended to drink it while covered in blankets to promote sweating.

2. Tincture:

- Preparation: Combine the dried leaves and flowers with a high-proof alcohol (usually vodka) in a jar in a ratio of 1:5 (herb to alcohol by weight to volume). Seal and store the jar in a cool, dark place for about 4-6 weeks, shaking it periodically. Strain the liquid through a fine mesh or cheesecloth into a dark bottle for storage.
- Usage: Tinctures are typically administered in small amounts (drops), diluted in water or tea.

3. Poultice:

- Application: For external use, a poultice made from the fresh or rehydrated dried leaves can be applied to the skin to help relieve muscle pain or inflammation. This is done by mashing the leaves into a paste and applying it directly to the affected area.

Safety and Considerations:

Toxicity Concerns: Boneset contains pyrrolizidine alkaloids, which can be toxic to the liver and carcinogenic if consumed in high quantities or over prolonged periods. It should be used with caution and not for extended periods.

Pregnancy and Nursing: Due to its constituents and potential toxicity, boneset should not be used during pregnancy or breastfeeding.

Interactions: Boneset may interact with other medications, especially those that affect liver function. It's important to consult with a healthcare provider before beginning any new herbal treatment, particularly if you are on medication or have existing health conditions.

Visnaga, Daucus visnaga

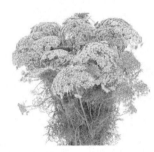

Composition:

- Primary Components: Contains khellin and visnagin, which are furanochromones that are thought to be responsible for its medicinal properties, including vasodilatory and bronchodilatory effects.
- Other Phytochemicals: Also contains flavonoids and volatile oils.

Visnaga, known for its distinct bitter and aromatic qualities, is more revered for its health benefits than its culinary uses. This herb acts as a potent muscle relaxer and has been a go-to remedy for the intense discomfort caused by kidney stones for ages. Modern studies have backed up its historical applications. Visnaga's component, khellin, has been the basis for creating exceptionally safe asthma medications. This plant is indigenous to North Africa and thrives in the wild across the Middle East and the Mediterranean region. It has also taken root in places like Australia and South America. Cultivated from seeds, visnaga is harvested before the tiny fruits fully mature at the end of summer.

Uses:

1. In 1946, an Egyptian pharmacologist discovered that visnaga, especially the chemicals khellin and visnagin, can significantly ease spasms in small bronchial and coronary arteries, as well as urinary passages. The effects on the bronchi can last up to six hours, and the plant is virtually free of side effects.

2. An age-old Egyptian solution for kidney stones, visnaga was even mentioned in the ancient Ebers Papyrus. It continues to be used for this purpose in Egypt, where it helps to lessen the agony of kidney stones by relaxing the ureter, allowing the stone to pass more comfortably into the bladder.

3. Due to its antispasmodic qualities, visnaga is now a recommended treatment for asthma, and it's even safe for kids. While it might not always halt an acute asthma attack, it can help in preventing them from happening again.

4. Visnaga has proven to be an effective treatment for various respiratory issues, including bronchitis, emphysema, and whooping cough.

5. It also helps with heart health by dilating coronary arteries, which improves blood flow to the heart muscle, thus relieving angina. However, it doesn't lower blood pressure.

6. In Andalusia, Spain, the locals have used the largest and finest visnaga seeds for dental hygiene, particularly teeth cleaning.

Preparation:

1. Tea (Infusion):

- Simple Preparation: Steep 1-2 teaspoons of dried visnaga seeds or fruits in a cup of boiling water for about 10 minutes. Strain before drinking.
- Dosage: This tea can be consumed 2-3 times a day, especially for treating urinary and respiratory conditions. The seeds can also be ground into a powder and used in similar ways.

2. Tincture:

- Preparation: Soak dried visnaga fruits or seeds in a mixture of alcohol and water (usually a ratio of 1:5) in a sealed jar. Keep the jar in a cool, dark place for 4-6 weeks, shaking it periodically. Strain the mixture into a clean bottle for storage.
- Usage: A typical dosage of the tincture might be a few drops added to water, taken several times per day.

3. Extracts:

- Commercial Extracts: Due to the specific active ingredients, such as khellin, it is common to use standardized commercial extracts to ensure consistent dosing, especially for clinical purposes like treating asthma.

Safety and Considerations:

Pregnancy and Nursing: Visnaga should not be used during pregnancy as it may lead to contractions or other complications. Its safety during breastfeeding is also not established.

Side Effects: Some of the compounds in visnaga, like khellin, can cause side effects such as nausea, dizziness, or sleep problems if taken in large doses or for prolonged periods.

Interactions: Due to its effects on the cardiovascular system, visnaga may interact with heart medications, especially those that affect heart rhythm or blood pressure. It's crucial to consult a healthcare provider before using visnaga, particularly if you are on any such medications.

Borage, Borago officinalis

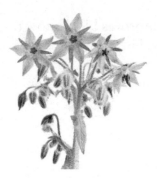

Composition:

- **Primary Components:** Contains gamma-linolenic acid (GLA), a type of Omega-6 fatty acid that's important for skin health and anti-inflammatory processes.
- **Other Phytochemicals:** Borage also includes mucilage, tannins, and flavonoids.

Borage, a common annual plant found in many gardens, is a magnet for bees who love its nectar and create delicious honey. This plant is easily recognized by its stiff white hairs covering its surface. It has succulent, hollow, and branched stems that can grow up to around 18 inches tall. The deep green, wrinkled leaves are arranged alternately, shaped like ovals with points, and measure about 3 inches in length and 1.5 inches in width. The underside of the lower leaves is also hairy, especially along the veins. The edges of the leaves are wavy, yet smooth.

The borage plant is adorned with striking blue, star-shaped flowers that feature black anthers arranged in a cone-like pattern at the center, often described as a beauty spot. These blooms start off pink and gradually turn blue, dangling in attractive clusters that eventually yield four brownish-black nutlets.

Uses:

1. You can munch on the leaves, flowers, dried stems, and seeds since they're all packed with nutrients. Enjoy the leaves fresh or cooked – toss them into salads or sauté them as a green. They have a fresh, cucumber-like taste, but it's best to eat them when they're young since the mature leaves can be a bit too fuzzy for some tastes.

2. The dried stems can add a unique flavor to dishes, and the seeds are loaded with gamma-linolenic acid (GLA), a type of Omega-6 that's good for you, although gathering them in significant amounts can be tricky.

3. Borage is great for balancing hormones and keeping your metabolism ticking. Regularly including borage in your meals can help smooth out your metabolism, ease PMS and menopausal symptoms, and regulate your menstrual cycle.

4. Feeling stressed? Borage can help calm you down. It's known to help balance cortisol levels, which can support your body's stress response and help with conditions like HPA-Dysfunction, sometimes known as Adrenal Fatigue.

5. The antioxidants in borage are like your body's personal defense team against aging and cancers caused by free radicals.

6. For those with an upset stomach or irritable bowel syndrome, borage can be quite soothing. It helps reduce inflammation in the gut, addresses gastritis, and other digestive issues. Plus, it aids digestion, stabilizes the stomach, and even has a gentle laxative effect.

7. If you're dealing with pneumonia, borage leaf and flower tea or tincture can help reduce symptoms, clear congestion, and help your body expel excess mucus. However, it's worth noting there might be better herbs out there for these symptoms.

8. Borage can also be used as a mouthwash or gargle to zap bacteria in the mouth and throat, preventing and treating sore throats and mouth sores.

9. Acting as a diuretic, borage helps eliminate extra water and toxins from your body and improves bladder function. It cleanses the bladder, fights off bacteria, and eases bladder infections, not to mention it can also soothe kidney inflammation and restore kidney health.

10. Nursing moms might find borage tea helpful for boosting milk production.

11. Lastly, a tea made from a mix of dried borage leaves and flowers can be a real lifesaver for hangovers.

Preparation:

1. Fresh Leaves and Flowers:

- Culinary Uses: Fresh borage leaves can be used in salads, or to garnish soups and drinks. The young leaves are preferable as older leaves can become rough and prickly.
- Preparation: Wash the leaves and flowers thoroughly before use. The leaves can be chopped finely and added to salads, or used as a wrap for finger foods.

2. Dried Herb:

- Tea: To make borage tea, steep 1-2 teaspoons of dried leaves or flowers in boiling water for about 10 minutes. This infusion can be drunk to exploit its medicinal properties.
- Storing Dried Herb: Dry the leaves or flowers in a dehydrator or in an airy, shaded spot, then store them in an airtight container away from light.

3. Oil:

- Borage Seed Oil: Typically extracted from the seeds, borage oil is rich in GLA and is commonly used as a dietary supplement.
- Usage: Borage oil can be used topically to moisturize the skin or taken orally as a supplement.

Safety and Considerations:

Potential Toxicity: Borage contains small amounts of pyrrolizidine alkaloids (PAs), which can be hepatotoxic and carcinogenic. However, the concentration is typically low in the leaves and flowers, and higher in parts not generally consumed.

Pregnancy and Breastfeeding: Due to the presence of PAs and limited research, it's best to avoid borage during pregnancy and breastfeeding.

Interactions: Borage oil can potentially interact with medications, especially those affecting blood clotting and those used to treat inflammation.

Dong Quai, Angelica sinensis

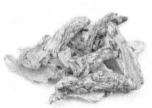

Composition:

- Primary Components: Contains phytoestrogens, coumarins (which have antispasmodic and vasodilatory effects), and essential oils.
- Other Phytochemicals: Also includes vitamins, minerals, and flavonoids that contribute to its overall health benefits.

In the heart of China, dong quai stands out as the go-to herbal remedy for women's health issues. Countless women incorporate it into their daily routine as a revitalizing elixir that helps balance their menstrual cycles and enrich their blood. Plus, it boosts blood flow. This herb is easily recognized by its unique, strong, yet sweet scent and is commonly added to meals in China, which is actually the preferred method to consume it for blood enrichment. Dong quai hails from China and Japan, and these days, it's mainly grown there. The finest roots come from China's Gansu province. They plant the seeds when spring arrives and harvest the roots come fall.

Uses

1. Studies in China dating back to the 1970s suggest that dong quai can help control the contractions of the uterus, which might be why it's effective for menstrual discomfort.

2. The root is known to support heart health and even acts as a blood thinner. This means it could potentially interact with blood-thinning medications.

3. Celebrated as a restorative in China, dong quai is consumed for conditions like "deficient blood," anemia, and anemia-related symptoms, such as a pale complexion, heart palpitations, and a general lack of energy.

4. It's great for regulating menstrual cycles, easing menstrual pain and cramps, and is especially beneficial for women who experience heavy periods and are at risk of anemia. However, if menstrual flow is intense, it's advisable to switch to other tonic herbs like nettle during that time. Dong quai is also known to support uterine health and may aid in addressing infertility.

5. As a "warming" herb, dong quai enhances circulation to the abdomen, hands, and feet. It's also good for digestive health and can be helpful in treating abscesses and boils.

Preparation:

1. Dried Root:

- Decoction: The most common way to prepare Dong Quai is by making a decoction. This involves simmering the dried root in water for 30-60 minutes. The longer you simmer it, the stronger the decoction will be.
- Powder: The dried root can also be ground into a powder and used in capsules or mixed into other forms such as teas or smoothies.

2. Tincture:

- Preparation: Soak the dried root in a mixture of alcohol and water (typically vodka or a similar spirit) for several weeks in a sealed container. This extracts the soluble compounds effectively. After the soaking period, strain the mixture and store the liquid in airtight containers.
- Tinctures are usually administered in small amounts (drops), which can be added to water or tea.

3. Tea:

- Simple Tea: For a lighter preparation, you can steep chopped or powdered Dong Quai root in boiling water for 15 to 20 minutes.
- Combination Herbal Teas: Often, Dong Quai is mixed with other herbs such as red raspberry leaf, nettle, or peppermint to enhance its flavor and medicinal properties.

Safety and Considerations:

Hormone Sensitivity: Due to its phytoestrogen content, Dong Quai should be used cautiously by individuals with hormone-sensitive conditions, such as breast, uterine, or ovarian cancers.

Pregnancy and Breastfeeding: Dong Quai is not recommended during pregnancy due to its potential to stimulate the uterus, which might lead to miscarriage. Its safety during breastfeeding is also not established.

Blood Thinning: Dong Quai has anticoagulant properties, which could increase the risk of bleeding, especially in people who are on blood-thinning medications like warfarin.

Bottle Gourd, Lagenaria siceraria

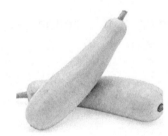

Composition:

- **Primary Components:** Bottle gourd is rich in dietary fiber, vitamin C, vitamin B, vitamin K, vitamin A, iron, folate, magnesium, and potassium.
- **Low in Calories:** It is also very low in saturated fat and cholesterol.

The bottle gourd, also referred to as the calabash, white-flowered gourd, or long melon, is commonly grown for its multipurpose fruit. When picked early, it's enjoyed as a vegetable. Once it's fully grown and dried, it can be hollowed out and used as a container or pipe. A member of the cucumber family, this plant is rarely found in the wild but thrives under cultivation. The vine can stretch over 15 feet long, bearing fruits with a pale green exterior and creamy interior, available in various shapes and sizes. Its stems are covered with long hairs that secrete a sticky substance. The leaves, which are either oval or heart-shaped, may have up to five shallow lobes. The solitary or paired white flowers bloom at night in the summer and close by morning.

Uses

1. It's primarily known to regulate blood sugar in diabetics. Some also value it for its heart-strengthening and calming properties. It's recognized for its anti-inflammatory, antioxidant, antibacterial, and analgesic qualities, along with being a tonic for the internal organs.

2. Regular consumption of bottle gourd can significantly reduce blood sugar levels in diabetic individuals. Just a couple of substantial bites with each meal can do the trick.

3. For those nagging headaches, a simple remedy is to mash its leaves into a poultice and apply it to the affected area on the head for relief.

4. Due to its antibacterial and anti-inflammatory properties, a poultice made from its boiled seeds can be applied to the skin to soothe irritations and infections. Wrap it with a clean cloth and keep it on to help lessen swelling and halt infection spread.

5. Research has indicated that the bottle gourd might be helpful in easing mild depression and enhancing memory, including for those with Alzheimer's Disease or age-related cognitive decline.

Preparation:

1. Fresh Gourd:

- Selection: Choose a young, firm bottle gourd with a pale green color. Older gourds can develop a bitter taste and tougher texture.
- Washing and Peeling: Wash the gourd thoroughly under running water, peel the outer skin, and then chop it into cubes or slices depending on your recipe.
- Cooking: Bottle gourd can be boiled, steamed, fried, or used as an ingredient in soups and stews.

2. Juicing:

- Juice Preparation: Grate the peeled gourd and press through a cheesecloth or use a juicer to extract the juice. It can be consumed directly or mixed with other fruit juices to enhance the flavor.
- Flavor Enhancements: Adding a bit of ginger, mint, or lemon juice can improve the taste of bottle gourd juice.

3. Dried Gourd:

- Uses: In addition to culinary uses, dried and hollowed bottle gourds are often used as utensils, musical instruments, or decorative objects.

Safety and Considerations:

Toxicity Warning: Bottle gourd juice occasionally turns out to be bitter and should be avoided since it may contain toxic substances that induce severe vomiting, diarrhea, and severe stomach discomfort. In severe situations, these toxic compounds can even be fatal.

Testing for Bitterness: Always taste a small piece of bottle gourd before using it to ensure it isn't bitter. Discard if it tastes bitter.

Allergic Reactions: Though rare, some people might be allergic to bottle gourd. Symptoms could include rashes, itching, or swelling.

Celery, Apium graveolens

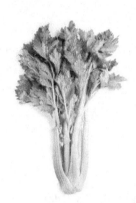

Composition:

- **Primary Components:** Rich in vitamin K, vitamin C, potassium, folate, and fiber.
- **Phytochemicals:** Contains luteolin, a flavonoid that can reduce inflammation and support neuron growth; and phthalides, which may help lower blood pressure.

Celery might be better known as a crunchy snack, but it's also got a history of being used for health issues like urinary troubles, rheumatic pain, and arthritis. The crunchy stalks and their seeds are packed with benefits. The seeds, in particular, are great for getting rid of unwanted substances in your body, especially if you're dealing with arthritis. They're also known to help you chill out a bit and ease digestion. Although the stalks aren't as potent in the health department, they still have their uses. Celery is a native plant around Europe and you can spot it in the wild along the coasts of England and Wales, as well as in marshy areas. The wild stuff is more aromatic than the celery we grow for our salads and soups. It's planted in the spring and harvested from the middle of summer to the fall season.

Uses:

1. Back in the '70s and '80s, studies figured out that the oils in celery can have a soothing effect on your nerves.

2. In 1995, researchers in India discovered that celery seeds are pretty good at protecting your liver. They might even help lower the fat in your blood. Some scientists in Iran in 2013 also noted that celery seeds could be a big help for folks with high blood pressure.

3. People have been growing celery for a super long time – at least 3,000 years. The ancient Egyptians were into it, and it was a thing in China around the 5th century BCE. It's been on the menu for ages, but it's also been a go-to remedy for various ailments.

4. These days, celery seeds are a go-to for treating conditions like rheumatic issues and gout. They're like a cleanup crew for your kidneys, helping to get rid of stuff your body doesn't need and balancing out your body's acid levels. They're also a buddy for your joints, boosting blood flow and helping to get rid of toxins.

5. Celery seeds have a bit of a diuretic effect and are pretty good at fighting off infections. They're a solid choice for dealing with bladder infections like cystitis because they help clean out your bladder and urinary tract.

6. Mixing up some celery and organic carrot juice gives you a super healthy drink that's perfect for tackling a bunch of long-term health problems.

7. Lastly, celery seeds can be a boon for respiratory issues like asthma and bronchitis. When you combine them with other herbs, they can also contribute to lowering blood pressure.

Preparation:

1. Fresh Celery:

- Selection: Choose crisp, tight bunches that snap easily when pulled; the leaves should be fresh and vibrant.
- Washing: Thoroughly wash celery to remove any dirt and potential chemical residues. It is one of the vegetables often treated with pesticides, so organic options are preferable for those trying to reduce their exposure.
- Slicing: Celery can be chopped into pieces for cooking or juiced. It is also commonly eaten raw.

2. Juicing:

- Juice Preparation: For a healthy drink, juice celery alone or with other fruits and vegetables like apple, carrot, and ginger for added flavor.
- Benefits: Celery juice is particularly popular in wellness communities for its purported benefits, such as detoxifying properties, improved digestion, and anti-inflammatory effects.

3. Dried Celery:

- Dehydrating: You can dry celery at low heat and then use it as a spice or store it for use in soups and stews.
- Powdered: Dried celery can also be ground into powder and used as a seasoning.

Safety and Considerations:

Allergic Reactions: Celery is one of the more common allergens, especially in Central Europe. People who are sensitive to birch pollen or mugwort may have a celery allergy, which can range from mild oral symptoms to severe reactions.

Pesticide Residue: Celery is often listed on the "Dirty Dozen" for vegetables with high pesticide residues, making organic choices preferable for those concerned about chemical exposure.

Medication Interactions: Due to its diuretic and blood pressure-lowering properties, celery might interact with diuretic and blood pressure medications.

Cabbage, Brassica oleracea

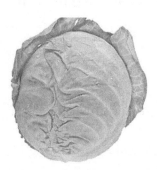

Composition:

•   **Primary Components:** Rich in vitamins C and K, fiber, and minerals like potassium and magnesium.
•   **Phytochemicals:** Contains glucosinolates, which may have cancer-preventive properties, and anthocyanins (in red cabbage) that have antioxidant effects.

Garden enthusiasts from coast to coast are well-acquainted with the humble cabbage, yet many might not be aware of its impressive medicinal qualities. This plant, which can be either biennial or perennial, develops into a spherical shape and can grow as tall as 8 feet (2.4m) when it reaches full maturity. Typically, cabbages are picked well before they get this big. Belonging to the Brassicaceae (Mustard) family, the cabbage has gray leaves and a robust stem. In springtime, it blooms with yellow four-petaled flowers. The leaves bunch up into a head by the end of the first summer. Cabbages come in shades of reddish-purple, green, or white, and regardless of the color, all share the same health-promoting properties outlined below.

Uses:

1. Cabbage is a staple, particularly in colder months, because it stores well in a root cellar. It's consumed both raw and cooked.

2. To alleviate sore, swollen breasts and mastitis, a cabbage leaf poultice does wonders. Remove the central vein and gently pound the leaf to release its healing sulfur compounds and juices. Place the battered leaf directly on the skin or inside the bra. Continue as needed until the situation gets better.

3. Cabbage leaves are excellent for cleaning wounds and warding off infections. They're also great at reducing swelling in achy joints and treating skin growths. Finely chop and mash the leaves to let out their beneficial juices, then warm them with minimal water. Use this warm mash as a poultice on the sore spots. It detoxifies and prevents bacterial growth while easing inflammation.

4. Cabbage is beneficial for digestive issues, thanks to its sulfur-rich makeup. When fermented into sauerkraut, its potency for aiding digestive troubles increases.

5. A concoction of sauerkraut juice with a splash of lemon juice can assist individuals in managing diabetes and maintaining stable blood sugar levels. This mix boosts digestion and the function of the pancreas.

6. To combat cancer, particularly those affecting the stomach, intestines, pancreas, and prostate, incorporate cabbage juice or sauerkraut juice into your routine twice a day. You can also eat finely chopped cabbage as your body allows. Both forms of cabbage are packed with compounds that are anti-cancerous and promote healing throughout the body.

Preparation:

1. Fresh Cabbage:

- Selection: Choose heads that feel heavy for their size with crisp, tightly packed leaves. The outer leaves should be free from major blemishes and the stem should appear freshly cut.
- Washing and Cutting: Wash the outer leaves thoroughly to remove any dirt or chemical residues. Peel off and discard the outer leaves, then slice the cabbage according to the recipe requirements—this could be shredding for coleslaw, chopping for stews, or keeping whole leaves for wraps.
- Cooking: Cabbage can be steamed, boiled, sautéed, or eaten raw. It's commonly used in salads, soups, stir-fries, and as a fermented product in dishes like sauerkraut and kimchi.

2. Fermented Cabbage (Sauerkraut/Kimchi):

- Preparation: For sauerkraut, finely slice the cabbage, mix it with salt, and pack it tightly in a jar so that the salt draws out the water and covers the cabbage. This should then be left to ferment at room temperature for several weeks. Kimchi involves a similar process but includes a variety of other ingredients like chili peppers, garlic, ginger, and sometimes fish sauce.
- Benefits: Fermentation enhances the digestibility and nutritional profile of cabbage, adding probiotics which are beneficial for gut health.

3. Juicing:

- Juice Preparation: Cabbage can also be juiced, often mixed with fruits like apples or carrots to improve its palatability.
- Consumption Tips: Cabbage juice is reputed to help with inflammation and gut health, including conditions like ulcers.

Safety and Considerations:

Goitrogens: Like other cruciferous vegetables, cabbage contains goitrogens, which can interfere with thyroid hormone production, especially if consumed in large quantities and particularly when raw.

Gas and Bloating: Due to its high fiber and sulfur content, some people may experience gas and bloating after eating cabbage, especially when it is eaten raw or fermented.

Burdock, Arctium lappa

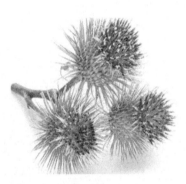

Composition:

- **Primary Components:** Rich in inulin, a type of soluble fiber that acts as a prebiotic, promoting gut health.
- **Other Nutrients:** Contains high levels of antioxidants, including phenolic acids, quercetin, and luteolin, and is also a good source of vitamins B6 and E, magnesium, potassium, iron, and manganese.

Burdock is widely recognized as a stellar herb for detoxifying the body, valued in both Western and Eastern herbal medicine practices. People often turn to it when dealing with health issues that stem from an accumulation of toxins, such as sore throats, skin problems like boils, rashes, and chronic skin conditions. The roots and seeds of burdock are celebrated for their waste-eliminating properties, with the roots being especially effective at removing heavy metals from the body. Native to Europe and Asia, burdock has adapted to temperate regions across the globe, including the U.S. It's cultivated in Europe and China, planted in spring from seeds, with the seeds harvested in summer and the whole plant collected at the height of the season.

Uses:

1. Studies from Germany in 1967 and Japan in 1986 discovered that polyacetylenes, predominantly in the fresh root, have antibacterial properties.

2. Burdock is known for its antibacterial and antifungal effects, it acts as a diuretic, helps in lowering blood sugar, and might even have anti-tumor benefits. The seeds are recently identified as anti-inflammatory, full of antioxidants, and liver-protective.

3. Burdock has traditionally been used for ailments like gout, fevers, and kidney stones. Culpeper in the 17th century praised the seeds for their ability to crush kidney stones and promote their expulsion through urine.

4. In both Western and Chinese herbal medicine, burdock seeds are utilized to detoxify the body during fevers and infections, including mumps and measles. The root is also used to help rid the body of waste in persistent skin and joint conditions.

5. Thanks to its diuretic, antibiotic, and slightly bitter qualities, burdock is particularly helpful for skin conditions linked to toxicity, such as acne, abscesses, localized infections, eczema, and psoriasis.

6. Burdock is rarely used on its own; it's often paired with other herbs like dandelion or yellow dock. These companions support the elimination process that burdock initiates in the tissues.

Preparation:

1. Fresh Root:

- Selection and Cleaning: Choose firm, unblemished burdock roots. Wash them thoroughly under running water to remove soil and debris. Scrubbing with a brush can help remove embedded dirt.
- Peeling: Peel the outer skin with a vegetable peeler to reveal the white inner flesh, which can darken upon exposure to air.
- Cooking: Burdock root can be sliced and added to stir-fries, soups, or stews. It can also be roasted or eaten raw in salads.

2. Dried Burdock:

- Tea Preparation: Dried burdock root can be steeped in boiling water to make a herbal tea. This is commonly consumed for its purported health benefits.

- Storing: Keep dried burdock root in a cool, dry place in an airtight container to preserve its potency.

3. Tincture:

- Making Tincture: Soak chopped fresh or dried root in alcohol, such as vodka, to extract the active compounds. This mixture should sit in a dark place for several weeks, shaken occasionally, then strained for use.
- Usage: Tinctures are typically used in small doses, often diluted in water.

Safety and Considerations:

Allergic Reactions: People who are sensitive to other members of the Asteraceae/Compositae family, such as chrysanthemums, daisies, or ragweed, may also be allergic to burdock.

Drug Interactions: Burdock may interact with blood thinners, diabetes medications, or diuretics due to its blood sugar lowering and diuretic effects.

Pregnancy and Breastfeeding: There is limited research on the safety of burdock use during pregnancy and breastfeeding, so it is best to avoid it during these times.

Calendula, Calendula officinalis

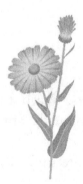

Composition:

- **Primary Components:** Contains flavonoids, carotenoids, and saponins, which contribute to its anti-inflammatory and antimicrobial properties.
- **Other Phytochemicals:** Also includes triterpenoids and polysaccharides, which are useful in promoting skin healing and health.

Calendula, also known as Pot Marigold, is typically a perennial member of the Aster/Daisy family but is commonly grown as an annual. It's not originally from North America, yet it thrives in many gardens, reseeds itself, and is quite simple to cultivate. It reaches heights of 12 to 24 inches, sporting either sprawling or upright stems. The plant has oblong, lance-shaped leaves that are hairy and range from 2 to 7 inches in length. These leaves might have smooth, wavy, or slightly toothed edges. Sporting yellow or orange blooms, Calendula features flower heads about 2 to 3 inches across with two layers of hairy bracts. In milder regions, it blooms all year. Some blossoms boast several layers of petals, while others have just one. Varieties with more resin and petals are often preferred for medicinal uses, and the plant produces small, curved seeds.

Uses:

1. You can munch on fresh Calendula flowers in salads or use them dried as a spice. They're a visual stand-in for saffron but don't expect the same flavor. Petal tea is a thing, too. The leaves are technically edible but tend to be too bitter for most tastes.

2. Calendula is kind to the skin, offering relief from a spectrum of skin woes, including pimples, sunburn, and rashes, even the ones babies get. Crushed leaves can be applied to small wounds, scrapes, bites, and skin annoyances for healing.

3. It's also a friend to slow-healing sores like ulcers and hemorrhoids, thanks to its use in creams, gels, or balms. It encourages quicker healing, firmer skin, and better hydration, all while fighting off microbes and bacteria.

4. Boosting your immune system and your skin's collagen is another Calendula perk. Whip up an anti-aging concoction with it and Cottonwood Buds in almond oil for a natural face cream alternative.

5. It's also a muscle relaxant, handy for easing spasms. Drinking Calendula tea can help with abdominal and menstrual cramps.

6. Speaking of menstrual discomfort, Calendula tea is your ally. It not only eases the pain but also helps kick-start your period, relaxes muscles, and improves circulation. Some even say it helps with hot flashes.

7. With its strong antibacterial properties, Calendula is excellent for oral health, tackling gingivitis, plaque, cavities, and other dental issues.

8. Digestive issues like intestinal colitis, GERD, esophageal irritation, stomach ulcers, and inflammatory bowel disease can all benefit from Calendula's soothing touch, as it eases inflammation and aids in healing.

9. Its anti-inflammatory abilities also make it a potential ally in the fight against cancer and in soothing the irritations from cancer treatments. It activates the lymphatic system to combat cancer cells and helps alleviate skin discomfort post-radiation therapy.

Preparation:

1. Infusion (Tea):

- Simple Tea Preparation: Steep 1-2 teaspoons of dried calendula flowers in a cup of boiling water for about 10 minutes. This tea can be used for drinking or as a rinse for skin and hair.
- Dosage: As a drink, calendula tea can be consumed 1-2 times daily. As a topical application, it can be used as needed on the skin or scalp.

2. Tincture:

- Alcohol Extraction: To make a calendula tincture, soak the dried flowers in a high-proof alcohol (like vodka) for 4-6 weeks. Strain the flowers out, and the remaining liquid is used as a concentrated form for topical application or internal use in diluted form.
- Usage: A few drops of the tincture can be applied to the skin or added to water and taken orally.

3. Topical Applications (Salve, Cream, Oil):

- Oil Infusion: Fill a jar with dried calendula flowers, cover with a carrier oil (such as olive oil or almond oil), and leave to infuse for about 4 weeks or gently heat for a few hours in a double boiler. Strain the flowers out and use the oil as a base for creams or as a skin soothing oil.
- Creams and Salves: Mix the infused oil with beeswax to make a salve or with other ingredients like shea butter to make a cream. These preparations are excellent for treating dry skin, rashes, and minor cuts and burns.

Safety and Considerations:

Allergies: People sensitive to other members of the Asteraceae family, such as daisies and ragweed, may also be allergic to calendula.

Pregnancy and Breastfeeding: The use of calendula is not well studied in pregnant or breastfeeding women, so it's best to use caution and consult a healthcare provider.

Interactions: Calendula is generally safe but can interact with sedative medications due to its mild sedative properties.

Wormwood, Artemisia absinthium

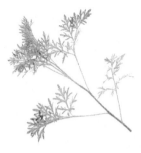

Composition:

- **Primary Components**: Contains thujone, a ketone and monoterpene that influences the nervous system and is toxic in high doses. It also includes other volatile oils, sesquiterpene lactones, and flavonoids which contribute to its bitter properties and medicinal effects.
- **Other Phytochemicals**: Wormwood is also rich in antioxidants and phenolic compounds.

Wormwood, known for its distinct lack of sweetness—hence the name absinthium—is a plant recognized for its robust effect on the digestive system, particularly the stomach and gallbladder. It's usually consumed in tiny amounts, with its potent bitter flavor playing a crucial role in its healing properties. Historically, wormwood was a key ingredient in vermouth, which gets its name from the German word for wormwood. This roadside herb is indigenous to Europe and now also thrives in central Asia, the eastern United States, and is cultivated globally in temperate zones. You can grow wormwood by planting seeds in the spring or splitting its roots in the fall, and you harvest the parts above ground come late summer.

Uses

1. Studies from the 1970s suggest that various components in wormwood, known for their bitterness, trigger the bitter taste receptors, which in turn stimulate the digestive system.

2. A 2007 study in Germany showed promising results for using wormwood to manage Crohn's disease, with 90% of participants seeing a halt in the recurrence of symptoms and a decrease in the need for potent anti-inflammatory steroids, alongside a reduction in depression.

3. Wormwood's essential oil, in particular, is believed to have a broad spectrum of health benefits, including protecting nerve cells, lifting mood, fighting bacteria and fungi, and combating malaria.

4. Wormwood is infamous for its use in absinthe, a once-popular addictive beverage in 19th-century France. Although flavored with wormwood oil, absinthe's toxicity came from its high thujone content—a nerve stimulant that's safe in small doses but dangerous when overconsumed.

5. For those suffering from sluggish digestion, wormwood can be a godsend. It boosts stomach acid and bile, enhancing digestion and nutrient absorption, which can be beneficial

for various conditions, including anemia. It also relieves gas and bloating and can gradually fortify the digestive system, particularly after a long illness.

6. Herbalists often turn to wormwood to clear out gut parasites, such as worms, amebic dysentery, and Shigella infections.

7. As a traditional remedy, wormwood serves as an effective insecticide and deterrent for bugs.

8. The plant's anti-inflammatory qualities make it a candidate for treating infections and it has been used occasionally as an antidepressant.

Preparation:

1. Tea (Infusion):

- Simple Preparation: Steep about 1/2 to 1 teaspoon of dried wormwood leaves in a cup of boiling water for 5-10 minutes. Due to its very bitter flavor, it's usually taken in small amounts.
- Dosage Caution: It's important to limit the amount of wormwood tea consumed; typically, it's recommended to drink no more than 3-4 cups per week, as excessive consumption can lead to adverse effects due to the thujone content.

2. Tincture:

- Alcohol Extraction: Wormwood can be soaked in alcohol to make a tincture, extracting the active compounds more effectively than water. This should be used sparingly, typically a few drops in water, due to the potent effects of the herb.
- Usage: Taken before meals, it can stimulate the appetite and aid digestion.

3. Wormwood Oil:

- Wormwood can also be processed into an essential oil, which should be used externally due to the high concentration of active substances. It's potent and must be diluted with a carrier oil before topical application.
- External Use: Used in aromatherapy and as an antiseptic for minor cuts and abrasions.

Safety and Considerations:

Thujone Toxicity: Thujone is neurotoxic and can cause seizures if consumed in high amounts. It's crucial to use wormwood under the guidance of a healthcare professional and not exceed recommended doses.

Pregnancy and Breastfeeding: Due to its potent effects and thujone content, wormwood should not be used during pregnancy or breastfeeding.
Wormwood may interact with medications, particularly those that affect the central nervous system. Its use with other sedative drugs should be carefully monitored.

Duration of Use: Long-term use of wormwood is not recommended due to the potential for neurotoxicity. Use should be limited to a few weeks at a time.

California Poppy, Eschscholzia californica

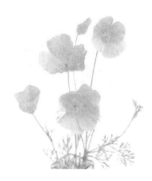

Composition:

- **Primary Components:** Contains alkaloids, including californidine and protopine, which are thought to contribute to its sedative and antispasmodic effects.
- **Other Phytochemicals:** Also rich in flavonoids, carotenoids, and other phenolic compounds that provide antioxidant benefits.

The California poppy, a member of the Papaveraceae family, is renowned for its calming and restorative properties, though it doesn't have the psychoactive or narcotic qualities found in certain other poppies. This plant is a native of Western North America and thrives in diverse environments such as coastal areas, foothills, valleys, and deserts, up to an elevation of 7000 feet. Also known as the Golden Poppy or Cup of Gold due to its vibrant golden hue, this plant can be an annual or a robust perennial, standing between half a foot to two feet tall with blue-green leaves that are compound and almost hairless.

The California poppy boasts striking flowers with bright orange to yellow petals, often with a darker orange at the center. Its seed capsules are cylindrical and pop open at the base when they're ripe, scattering the seeds up to six feet away. These seeds are small, round, and typically gray to brown when fully mature.

Uses:

1. It's a natural diuretic, eases muscle spasms, soothes pain, encourages sweating, and has a calming effect. It's non-addictive and can even assist with easing off opiates, likely interacting with GABA receptors. The whole plant has medicinal uses, but the root packs the most punch.

2. As a gentle sedative, the California poppy is particularly good for treating bedwetting in kids. It helps with sleep issues, anxiety, and stress. The sap has a somewhat numbing effect, making it great for toothaches. It's not a downer for your nervous system and is gentler than its opium cousin. Best taken before bed, it can help you catch some Z's and is also an antispasmodic.

3. For those grappling with mental health challenges, California poppy can help stabilize thought processes, and it's gentle enough for kids. It doesn't have a narcotic effect but rather soothes the mind and aids in restoring normalcy. It's particularly effective for anxiety and PTSD.

4. If you're looking to stop lactation, a wash made from California Poppy Tea using the roots can be applied to the breasts to halt milk production swiftly.

Preparation:

1. Tea (Infusion):

- Simple Preparation: Steep 1-2 teaspoons of dried California poppy flowers and leaves in a cup of boiling water for about 10 minutes. This herbal tea can be drunk before bedtime to help induce relaxation and improve sleep quality.
- Dosage: It's generally recommended to drink this tea 30 minutes before bedtime for best results.

2. Tincture:

- Alcohol Extraction: Soak the dried aerial parts of the California poppy in a mixture of alcohol and water (usually vodka or a similar spirit) for several weeks to makehe soaking period, strain the liquid and store it in a dark bottle.
- Usage: Tinctures are more concentrated than teas and are typically used in smaller doses, such as a few drops in water, particularly before bedtime. a tincture. This method extracts the active compounds effectively. After t

3. Topical Application:

- Infused Oil: You can infuse the dried flowers in a carrier oil (like olive or almond oil) for several weeks, and then use the strained oil topically for its analgesic properties on areas affected by pain or inflammation.

Safety and Considerations:

Contraindications: While generally considered safe, California poppy should not be used in conjunction with strong sedatives or other CNS depressants due to potential additive effects.

Pregnancy and Breastfeeding: There is insufficient data on its safety during pregnancy and breastfeeding, so it is best avoided during these times.

Allergic Reactions: As with any plant, some individuals may experience allergic reactions, particularly those who are sensitive to other members of the poppy family.

Sweet Annie, Artemisia annua

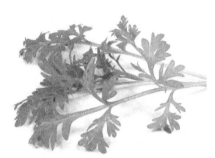

Composition:

- **Primary Components:** Contains artemisinin, a sesquiterpene lactone, which is effective against malaria and has shown potential in cancer therapy research.
- **Other Phytochemicals:** Also rich in flavonoids and essential oils, which contribute to its anti-inflammatory and antimicrobial effects.

Before the 1970s, sweet Annie was simply considered one of many Artemisia plants, but it was valued in Chinese traditional medicine for fighting malaria. Subsequent in-depth studies revealed that sweet Annie and its primary component, artemisinin, possess potent antimalarial properties with minimal adverse effects. Artemisinin swiftly emerged as the go-to remedy for severe malaria globally and remains a preferred option for many cases of the disease today. Sweet Annie thrives in grassy areas and clearings across Vietnam, Japan, China, Russia, and North America, and is specifically cultivated in eastern China. This herb can be propagated by sowing seeds in the spring or dividing its rootstock come fall, and it's typically harvested in the summer before it blooms.

Uses:

1. In-depth research in China during the 1980s established sweet Annie's main active ingredient as a formidable foe against the malaria-causing Plasmodium parasite, which mosquitoes transmit to humans.

2. Lab studies indicate that sweet Annie may exhibit significant anti-cancer effects, possibly triggering cell death and hindering the growth of blood vessels. While clinical trials are pending, there are claims of its effectiveness, particularly against breast cancer and leukemia. Additionally, synthetic compounds inspired by artemisinin are under investigation as potential cancer treatments.

3. The earliest reference to sweet Annie dates back to a Chinese manuscript from 168 BCE, where it was recommended for "dispelling and soothing the heat of summer."

4. Known for its cool, bitter flavor, sweet Annie is utilized for heat-induced ailments, notably those presenting with fever, headaches, dizziness, and feelings of tightness in the chest. It's a go-to for persistent fevers, night sweats, and morning chills and has been a traditional cure for heat-related nosebleeds.

5. For millennia, sweet Annie has been a remedy for the fever and chills of malaria, and nowadays, artemisinin is widely used as an antimalarial agent. While artemisinin helps in preventing malaria and ensuring rapid recovery, resistance to the drug is emerging. The whole plant might also be used for treating and preventing malaria, but it requires high doses.

Preparation:

1. Tea (Infusion):

- Simple Preparation: Steep 1-2 teaspoons of dried Sweet Annie leaves in a cup of boiling water for 10-15 minutes. This tea can be used for various medicinal purposes, including reducing fever and inflammation.
- Dosage: Drinking the tea 1-2 times a day can help alleviate symptoms of various ailments; however, it should be used with caution due to the potency of its active compounds.

2. Tincture:

- Alcohol Extraction: Soak the dried leaves in alcohol (typically vodka) for several weeks to make a tincture. This extracts the active compounds more effectively than water alone.
- Usage: Tinctures are typically used in small amounts, usually a few drops in water, and taken once or twice daily.

3. Essential Oil:

- Steam Distillation: The leaves and flowering parts can be subjected to steam distillation to produce an essential oil, which concentrates the plant's volatile compounds.
- Topical Application: The oil should be diluted with a carrier oil and can be applied to the skin to utilize its anti-inflammatory and antimicrobial properties.

Safety and Considerations:

Pregnancy and Breastfeeding: Sweet Annie is not recommended for use during pregnancy as it can cause contractions. Its safety for nursing infants is unknown.

Drug Interactions: Artemisinin can interact with other medications, especially those that affect liver enzymes which metabolize drugs.

Long-Term Use: Long-term use of Sweet Annie, particularly high doses, is not recommended due to potential liver toxicity.

Allergic Reactions: As with any herbal product, some people may develop an allergic reaction to Sweet Annie, particularly if they are sensitive to other plants in the Asteraceae family.

Carolina Geranium, Geranium carolinianum

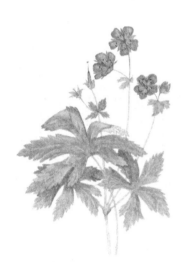

Composition:

- **Primary Components:** Contains tannins, which are responsible for its astringent properties, and flavonoids, which contribute antioxidant benefits.
- **Other Phytochemicals:** Also includes polyphenolic acids and various essential oils that may have anti-inflammatory and antimicrobial effects.

Carolina Geranium, also known as Carolina Cranesbill or Wild Geranium, is a plant native to the United States, Canada, and Mexico. It thrives in less fertile soils, including clay and limestone environments, and is commonly spotted along roadsides, in neglected fields, and on farms. This herbaceous plant is either a winter annual or biennial, standing less than a foot tall. It's called "cranesbill" due to the fruit's resemblance to a bird's beak. Its palmate leaves, which are 1 to 2.5 inches wide, have 5 to 7 lobes, each deeply toothed and split further, and are covered in fine hairs. The stems are pinkish-red, erect, and hairy. From April to July, you'll find white, pink, or lavender flowers in clusters, each with five sepals and petals. In autumn, the fruits, about half an inch long with a longer style, mature and feature pitted seeds. The plant has a shallow taproot system.

Uses

1. You can eat Carolina Geranium raw, cook it, or brew it into a tea. The roots are a bit tough, so boiling them for 10 minutes softens them up. Plus, the water you boil them in makes a soothing tea for upset stomachs. The leaves can be quite bitter due to their high tannin content, but using them when they're young or changing the boiling water halfway through cooking can help with that. People often enjoy the tea with a dash of milk and cinnamon to make it tastier.

2. The whole plant acts as an astringent because it's packed with tannins, which can help to halt bleeding by tightening tissues. Applying a poultice made from the root or leaves to damp wounds can help dry them out, and it's great in skin salves for healing.

3. If you have a sore throat, the root can be quite comforting, and it might even fight off viruses.

4. When turned into a tincture, the Carolina Geranium root contains compounds like geraniin and hyperin, which have shown activity against Hepatitis B.

5. A tea brewed from the root is perfect for settling an upset stomach and calming diarrhea.

6. If you're dealing with a canker sore, rinsing with Carolina Geranium tea or applying a root poultice can dry it out and help it heal quickly thanks to the root's astringent properties.

Preparation:

1. Tea (Infusion):

- Simple Preparation: Steep 1-2 teaspoons of dried Carolina Geranium leaves in a cup of boiling water for about 10 minutes. This herbal tea can be used to leverage the plant's astringent properties for treating mild digestive disorders and as a gargle for sore throats.
- Dosage: Consuming the tea once or twice a day can help with gastrointestinal discomfort and oral health.

2. Tincture:

- Alcohol Extraction: To make a tincture, soak the dried leaves and possibly roots in alcohol (usually vodka) for several weeks. This method extracts a concentrated form of the active compounds.
- Usage: Typically used in small amounts, a few drops of the tincture can be added to water and consumed to help with digestive issues and skin conditions.

3. Topical Application:

- Poultice: Fresh leaves can be crushed to form a poultice and applied to the skin to help soothe irritations and minor wounds. The astringent properties help tighten the skin and reduce inflammation.

Safety and Considerations:

Allergies: As with any plant, there's a risk of allergic reactions, particularly if you have allergies to other members of the Geranium family.

Pregnancy and Breastfeeding: There is limited research on the safety of Carolina Geranium during pregnancy and breastfeeding. It is advisable to avoid use during these times.

Interaction with Medications: Given its astringent properties, Carolina Geranium may interact with medications, especially those that affect blood clotting and gastrointestinal function.

Astragalus, Astragalus membranaceus

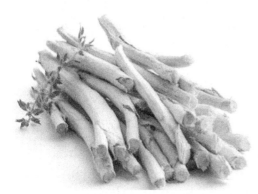

Composition:

- Primary Components: Contains saponins, flavonoids, and polysaccharides, which contribute to its immune-boosting and anti-inflammatory effects.
- Other Phytochemicals: Also includes various amino acids, trace minerals, and other compounds that support its traditional health claims.

Astragalus might be a big deal in China as a go-to health booster, but it's still flying under the radar in the West. Over in China, they've been tapping into the power of the huang qi root for ages. It's got a nice sweet flavor and works like a charm to pep up young, active folks by giving them more energy and helping them shake off the chill. Plus, it's a team player, often mixed with other herbs to get your blood in tip-top shape. This plant calls Mongolia and parts of China home, loves a sunny spot in sandy soil, and is planted either when spring kicks in or when autumn rolls around. Once the plants hit the four-year mark, it's time to collect those roots in the fall.

Uses:

1. The word from China is that astragalus can help you pee more, might take your blood pressure down a notch, and could even help you last longer when you're pushing yourself. A study in 2012 showed that taking 5 grams of the root daily could keep kidney disease from getting worse and hold off dialysis.

2. Over in the States, scientists are looking at how astragalus might get the immune system back on track for cancer patients. It seems that when folks are dealing with the rough ride of chemo or radiation, adding astragalus to the mix could help them bounce back quicker and stick around longer.

3. If you're on the younger side and need a pick-me-up, astragalus might even beat out ginseng. In China, they believe it cranks up the wei qi, which is like a protective vibe just under your skin, making you better at handling stuff like cold weather. It's also got a rep for cranking up your immune system and giving you a solid boost in the stamina department.

Barbara Parrish

4. Astragalus is also good for when you're sweating buckets or feeling puffed up with water. It gets your blood moving to the surface and is a buddy to your kidneys, keeping them from getting roughed up.

5. It's not your go-to for when you're down with something fierce, but astragalus has a knack for dealing with viral stuff like the common sniffles.

6. It's also got uses for when things are a bit out of place inside, like a droopy uterus, and is pretty handy for stopping uterine bleeding. Often, it's paired with *dong quai* to make a blood tonic that's great for anemia.

Preparation:

1. Decoction:
- Simple Preparation: To make an Astragalus decoction, add 10-30 grams of dried sliced root to about one liter of water. Bring it to a boil and then simmer for 30 minutes to a few hours to extract the deep-rooted benefits from the hard root slices.
- Dosage: This decoction can be consumed daily, typically 1-2 cups, as part of a health regimen to boost immunity and energy.

2. Tincture:
- Alcohol Extraction: Soak the dried root in alcohol (usually vodka) for 4-6 weeks to make a tincture, shaking the mixture periodically. This extracts the soluble compounds effectively.
- Usage: The tincture can be used in small doses (a few drops up to three times a day), often diluted in water or tea, especially during times when extra immune support is needed.

3. Powder:
- Ground Root: The dried root can also be ground into a fine powder and used in capsules or added to smoothies, soups, and other dishes for an easy boost of its beneficial properties.
- Consumption: Typically, 1-3 grams of the powder can be used daily, depending on the desired effects and personal tolerance.

Safety and Considerations:

Autoimmune Diseases: Because Astragalus stimulates the immune system, it should be used with caution in individuals with autoimmune diseases, as it could potentially exacerbate symptoms.

Medication Interactions: Astragalus may interfere with drugs that suppress the immune system and could also affect blood sugar levels and blood pressure; thus, it should be used cautiously by those on related medications.

Pregnancy and Breastfeeding: Due to limited research on its use during pregnancy and breastfeeding, it is best to avoid Astragalus in these situations unless directed by a healthcare provider.

Chamomile, Matricaria chamomilla

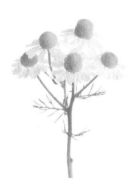

Composition:

- Primary Components: Contains flavonoids such as apigenin, which is known for its calming effects. It also includes essential oils like bisabolol and matricin, which contribute to its anti-inflammatory and healing properties.
- Other Phytochemicals: Chamomile is rich in antioxidants, which help combat oxidative stress and may contribute to overall health benefits.

Chamomile is a widely appreciated and beneficial herb known for its soothing qualities and sedative effects. It belongs to the Asteraceae or Daisy family and boasts daisy-like blooms with a distinctive hollow, cone-shaped center. The center is a bright yellow, encircled by 10 to 20 white petals that curve downward. Each flower sits atop its own stem, which helps in distinguishing chamomile from other similar plants. The easiest way to identify chamomile is to pick a bit of the flower and gently crush it between your fingers, releasing its subtly fruity aroma. Chamomile is a hardy plant that grows in the wild but can also be cultivated in your garden, preferring sunny spots with soil that drains well. It's not a fan of too much heat or drought.

There are two primary types of chamomile: German (Matricaria chamomilla) and English. They share many medicinal benefits but can be told apart by their foliage. German chamomile has slender, hairy leaves that are finely cut (bipinnate), while English chamomile leaves are broader and smoother. German chamomile also has a somewhat feathery stem, whereas the English variety does not. Depending on its environment, chamomile can reach heights of 2 to 3 feet.

Uses:

1. Chamomile is most commonly enjoyed as a tea, but it's also available as a tincture or in dried capsule form.

2. It's great for easing muscle cramps, including those in the digestive tract, which makes it a go-to remedy for stomach aches, indigestion, gastritis, bloating, Crohn's disease, and irritable bowel syndrome.

3. For eye discomfort, a chamomile eyewash can be made with 5 to 10 drops of tincture in boiled and cooled water, or by brewing a strong tea. This can help with eye strain and infections.

4. To alleviate congestion, try a steam treatment. Add a couple of teaspoons of chamomile petals to boiling water and breathe in the steam to loosen mucus. Alternatively, add a few drops of Chamomile Essential Oil to a vaporizer for overnight use.

5. Chamomile's antispasmodic properties can help relax muscles and ease body aches.

6. Drinking a cup of chamomile tea before bed or during nighttime can promote better sleep. If you need extra help, consider using a tincture.

7. For allergic reactions, like itchy skin or eczema, Chamomile Essential Oil, which has been altered through steam distillation to have anti-allergenic properties, can be diluted in a carrier oil for direct skin application or inhaled.

Preparation:

1. Tea (Infusion):

- Simple Preparation: To make chamomile tea, steep 1-2 teaspoons of dried chamomile flowers in a cup of boiling water for about 5-10 minutes. The longer you steep, the stronger the infusion will be.
- Dosage: Chamomile tea can be consumed several times a day to relieve stress, aid sleep, or reduce inflammation. It's gentle enough for frequent use.

2. Tincture:

- Alcohol Extraction: Soak dried chamomile flowers in alcohol (usually vodka) for a few weeks to create a tincture. This method concentrates the active ingredients for more potent therapeutic effects.
- Usage: Tinctures are generally used in small doses, often just a few drops in water, several times a day as needed for issues like anxiety or gastrointestinal discomfort.

3. Topical Applications:

- Oil or Cream: Infuse chamomile flowers in a carrier oil like sweet almond or olive oil for several weeks, then strain. The resulting oil can be used directly on the skin or as a base for creams and salves to treat skin irritations and inflammations.
- Compress: A chamomile tea compress (soaked cloth in cooled tea) can be applied to areas of skin irritation, sunburn, or under the eyes to reduce puffiness.

Safety and Considerations:

Allergies: Chamomile belongs to the same family as ragweed, marigolds, and daisies. People allergic to these plants might also be allergic to chamomile.

Pregnancy and Breastfeeding: While generally considered safe in small amounts, chamomile should be used cautiously during pregnancy due to potential effects on the uterus. See a medical professional before using.

Drug Interactions: Chamomile may interact with sedative medications and blood thinners. If you are taking any prescription medications, discuss with a healthcare provider before adding chamomile to your routine.

Deadly Nightshade, Atropa belladonna

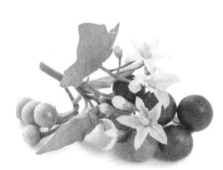

Composition:

- Primary Components: Contains alkaloids like atropine, scopolamine (hyoscine), and hyoscyamine, which are anticholinergic (they block acetylcholine, a neurotransmitter that affects the central and peripheral nervous system).
- Toxic Effects: All parts of the plant are toxic, with the berries being particularly dangerous due to their appealing appearance and potentially lethal content.

Despite its ominous reputation as a toxic plant, deadly nightshade actually plays a valuable role in both traditional and modern medicine when used responsibly. Its active ingredients are utilized in mainstream healthcare, for instance, to widen pupils during eye exams and to serve as a numbing agent. In the realm of herbal treatments, deadly nightshade is commonly recommended to soothe bowel cramps and to manage peptic ulcers. Originating from Europe, western Asia, and North Africa, this plant is now grown globally, favoring limestone-rich soil in wooded and open environments. The leaves are typically gathered in the summertime, while the root is harvested starting in the fall of its first year.

Uses:

1. Deadly nightshade once had a mystical reputation, thought to aid witches in flight. Its alternate name "belladonna" hints at its historical use by Italian women who applied it to enlarge their pupils, enhancing their allure.

2. Historically, deadly nightshade has been employed for its ability to ease tension in swollen body parts, particularly the stomach and bowels, alleviating colic and discomfort. It also aids

in treating peptic ulcers by cutting down on stomach acid and easing spasms in the urinary tract.

3. The plant has also been used to alleviate symptoms of Parkinson's disease, helping to lessen tremors and stiffness, while also improving speech and movement.

4. With its muscle-relaxing and anesthetic qualities, deadly nightshade is valuable in mainstream medicine, particularly for procedures requiring a reduction in digestive or respiratory secretions.

Safety and Considerations:

Extreme Toxicity: Belladonna is one of the most toxic plants known; ingestion of small quantities can be fatal. Symptoms of poisoning include dilated pupils, sensitivity to light, blurred vision, tachycardia, loss of balance, staggering, headache, rash, dry mouth and throat, slurred speech, urinary retention, constipation, confusion, hallucinations, delirium, and convulsions.

Medical Supervision Required: Due to its potency and risk, belladonna should never be used without medical supervision. Misuse can lead to poisoning or death.

Antidote Availability: Atropine, ironically also derived from belladonna, is used as an antidote for organophosphate poisoning (found in certain insecticides), which shows the complexity and danger of its active compounds.

Chickweed, Stellaria media

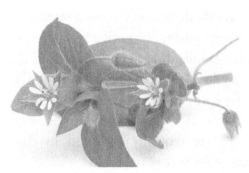

Composition:

•   Primary Components: Contains saponins, which have been shown to have anti-inflammatory properties, as well as flavonoids, vitamins C and A, and minerals like magnesium, calcium, potassium, and zinc.
•   Other Phytochemicals: Also includes coumarins and triterpenoids.

Chickweed is a yearly herb from the Caryophyllaceae, or Pink, family. This plant has found a second home across many regions in North America and is often called common chickweed to set it apart from similar-named species. Other nicknames include winterweed, maruns, starweed, and chickenwort. It's a favorite for feeding chickens and can grow anywhere between 2 to 20 inches tall. It tends to spread out, blanketing the ground it grows on. The flowers are petite, white, and star-like, while the oval leaves boast smooth edges with a slight frill and cupped tips.

Uses

1. You can eat the leaves, stems, and flowers either raw or cooked.

2. Brewing a tea or making a tincture from chickweed can help soothe arthritis pain and inflammation. A strong tea added to bathwater can also ease discomfort, particularly in the knees and feet.

3. For those dealing with the itchy rash of roseola, a poultice of mashed chickweed leaves can calm the itchiness and discomfort. Adding a potent tea to your bath is also beneficial.

4. Chickweed concoctions, like salves or poultices, are great for calming skin issues like itches, rashes, varicose veins, hives, dermatitis, and eczema. If you have a larger area to treat, mix it into your bathwater.

5. It's a powerful detoxifier and blood cleanser, pulling toxins from the body in cases of blood poisoning, tetanus, or toxins entering through wounds.

6. Applying chickweed as a poultice or salve can help alleviate the pain and tingling from misfiring surface nerves.

7. Drinking chickweed tea can ease constipation, but go easy on the brew as it's quite a strong laxative. While it can relieve digestive pain, it doesn't cure the root cause.

Preparation:

1. Fresh Plant Juice:
   - Simple Preparation: Fresh chickweed can be juiced or crushed to extract the liquid, which can be used fresh on skin irritations or taken internally for its vitamin and mineral content.
   - Dosage: Consume immediately after preparation to benefit from its fresh enzymes and nutrients.

2. Tea (Infusion):
   - Steeping: To make chickweed tea, steep about 1-2 teaspoons of fresh or dried chickweed in a cup of boiling water for about 10 minutes. This method is good for extracting its beneficial properties to soothe respiratory or digestive ailments.
   - Frequency: Can be drunk two to three times a day, particularly during episodes of coughs or colds to benefit from its mucilaginous properties.

3. Salve (Topical Application):
   - Oil Infusion: Infuse dried or fresh chickweed in a carrier oil like olive oil for several weeks (or gently heat for a few hours), then strain. Mix the infused oil with beeswax to make a salve. This can be applied to eczema, rashes, and other skin irritations.

- Use: Apply directly to the skin as needed to soothe and heal.

4. Tincture:

- Alcohol Extraction: Soak dried chickweed in alcohol for several weeks to make a tincture, which concentrates its medicinal properties.
- Usage: Use a few drops in water, taken 1-2 times daily, to support overall health and soothe internal inflammations.

Safety and Considerations:

Allergies: As with any plant, some individuals may be allergic to chickweed, especially those with sensitivities to other plants in the Caryophyllaceae family.

Pregnancy and Breastfeeding: There is limited research on the effects of chickweed during pregnancy and breastfeeding, so it is best to use it with caution or consult a healthcare provider.

Drug Interactions: Given chickweed's diuretic properties, it could potentially interact with diuretic medications or those affecting electrolyte balance.

Neem, Azadirachta indica

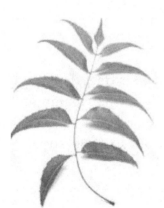

Composition:

- Primary Components: Contains nimbin, nimbinen, nimbolide, nimandial, ninbinene, and other compounds which contribute to its bitter taste and medicinal properties.
- Other Phytochemicals: Rich in antioxidants, fatty acids (in the oil), and similar bioactive compounds that provide anti-inflammatory, antifungal, and antipyretic effects.

Neem holds a prestigious spot in the world of Indian and traditional Ayurvedic health practices. Its leaf extracts are commonly employed to soothe various ailments including asthma, eczema, diabetes, and rheumatism. Neem oil, too, is a popular remedy for hair care, tackling head lice, and soothing irritated skin. Studies suggest that neem might be effective as both an insect repellent and a form of birth control. The tree is also celebrated for its air-purifying qualities and is a common sight across India. Originating from regions like Iran, Pakistan, India, and Sri Lanka, the neem tree is a familiar presence in forests and along roadways, offering shade. Its presence has spread to other warm climates such as Malaysia, Indonesia, Australia, and West Africa, where it has become naturalized. Neem grows from seeds and its leaves and seeds are collected year-round for various uses.

Uses:

1. Current studies show neem oil to possess anti-inflammatory and antibacterial properties, and it seems to also reduce fever and blood sugar levels to some extent.

2. In-depth research has revealed that the limonoid compounds known as azadirachtins in neem have insect-repelling properties and can disrupt feeding and growth in pests. These compounds are also associated with the tree's potential in fighting malaria.

3. Findings suggest that both neem leaves and oil can help regulate blood sugar, offering potential benefits for managing or postponing the onset of type 2 diabetes.

4. In India, the neem tree is often seen as a "village pharmacy," with all its parts having medicinal value. Its bark, known for its bitterness and astringency, is used in treating hemorrhoids. Neem leaves are used in various forms to combat issues like malaria, ulcers, and worms, and are also applied directly to skin conditions. Additionally, the leaf juice is used for eye conditions like night blindness and conjunctivitis, while the twigs serve as natural toothbrushes that support gum health.

5. Neem oil, extracted from seeds, is a go-to for hair care and has strong antifungal and antiviral properties, warding off conditions like scabies and ringworm. It's also crafted into treatments for head lice and various skin disorders including eczema, psoriasis, and even leprosy. However, those trying to conceive should steer clear of neem oil as it can impact fertility in both men and women.

Preparation:

1. Neem Tea:

- Simple Preparation: Boil a handful of dried neem leaves in water for about 5-10 minutes. Strain the leaves out and drink the tea for internal health benefits, such as blood purifying and immune-boosting effects.
- Dosage: Drink 1 cup of neem tea up to twice daily. Be cautious with consumption due to its strong effects, particularly on the liver and kidneys.

2. Neem Oil:

- Extraction: Neem oil is extracted from the seeds of the neem tree and is widely used for its pesticidal and medicinal properties. It can be applied topically but should be diluted with a carrier oil (like coconut or olive oil) to prevent irritation.
- Use: Apply diluted neem oil to the skin to treat acne, fungal infections, and even head lice.

3. Neem Paste:

- Creating Paste: Crush fresh or dried neem leaves with a little water to form a paste. This can be used as a skin mask or for healing skin ailments.
- Application: Apply the paste directly to the skin to address conditions like eczema, psoriasis, and ringworm.

4. Neem Chewing Sticks:

- Traditional Dental Care: In many parts of India, thin branches or twigs of the neem tree are used as natural toothbrushes. Chewing on these sticks helps to prevent dental decay, gum inflammation, and whitens teeth.

Safety and Considerations:

Pregnancy and Breastfeeding: Neem can have contraceptive properties and is advised against during pregnancy as it might lead to miscarriage or harm fetal development.

Internal Use Risks: Ingesting neem oil can be toxic; neem tea should be consumed in moderation as excessive intake can harm the liver and kidneys.

Allergic Reactions: Some people might be allergic to neem. Always test a small amount on your skin before widespread use.

Chicory, Cichorium intybus

Composition:

• Primary Components: Contains high levels of inulin, a type of soluble fiber that acts as a prebiotic to support healthy gut bacteria. It also has sesquiterpene lactones, which contribute to its bitter taste and are thought to have anti-inflammatory properties.

• Other Phytochemicals: Rich in antioxidants, including polyphenols and flavonoids.

The chicory plant, a member of the Aster/Daisy Family, can be either an annual or biennial. It has its origins in Eurasia but has spread across North America, where it's often classified as an invasive species in numerous areas. This plant goes by various names, including blue daisy, blue dandelion, blue sailors, blue weed, coffeeweed, cornflower, succory, wild bachelor's buttons, wild endive, and horseweed. It's sometimes mistaken for Curly Endive (Cichorium endivia), which is a relative that's also referred to as chicory. You can spot chicory by its distinctive purple blooms. It has stiff stems with hairy portions near the bottom. Its rough, toothed leaves resemble those of a dandelion, with the lower leaves being hairy and reaching up to 8 inches long. Both the stems and leaves ooze a white latex if they're broken.

Chicory can grow between 1 to 3 feet tall and features multiple flower heads that are about 1 to 1 1/2 inches across, typically grouped in twos or threes. The flowers, usually light blue-purple and occasionally pink or white, blossom from July to October. They have two layers of petals with jagged tips and tend to open in the morning, closing up as the day heats up. The plant is anchored by a thick, bitter taproot.

Uses

1. The roots and seeds of chicory can help get rid of worms and other parasites in your gut, and they have antibacterial, antifungal, and liver-protecting properties. There's ongoing research into using chicory roots in cancer treatment. The flowers and leaves are also beneficial for health and act as a gentle diuretic.

2. The fresh root's milky juice, much like that of Wild Lettuce, contains compounds called lactucin and lactucopicrin. These have calming and pain-relieving effects, akin to ibuprofen. It's best to use this latex directly or dry it for extraction in alcohol or oil rather than water, as they are sesquiterpene lactones.

3. Alcoholic extracts from chicory roots can get rid of intestinal worms and even attack the protozoan that causes cerebral malaria, Plasmodium falciparum. The roots' lactucin and lactucopicrin content have anti-malarial properties.

4. Using chicory leaf in a tincture, powder, or as part of a whole-plant alcohol extract can help manage insulin levels, encourage insulin production, and reduce blood sugar levels.

5. A coffee or tea brewed from chicory roots can aid in addressing digestive issues and ulcers.

6. For topical applications, you can wash skin blemishes with an infusion made from chicory leaves or apply crushed leaves as a poultice to inflamed areas. This has been shown to be effective by many.

Preparation:

1. Roasted Chicory Root:
   - Preparation for Coffee Substitute: The roots of the chicory plant can be harvested, cleaned, chopped, dried, and then roasted until brown. Once roasted, they can be ground and brewed just like coffee.
   - Use: Chicory root coffee can be enjoyed on its own or mixed with regular coffee. It is naturally caffeine-free, making it a popular coffee substitute.

2. Chicory Tea:

- Simple Tea Preparation: Steep about 1-2 teaspoons of dried chicory root or leaves in hot water for about 10 minutes.
- Benefits: Chicory tea is consumed for digestive benefits and as a liver tonic due to its detoxifying properties.

3. Chicory Leaves:

- Salads and Cooking: Young chicory leaves can be eaten raw in salads, while older leaves are typically cooked to reduce their bitterness. They can be sautéed with garlic and olive oil or added to soups and stews.
- Nutritional Value: High in vitamins and minerals, chicory leaves are a nutritious addition to meals.

4. Chicory Tincture:

- Alcohol Extraction: A tincture made from chicory root can be prepared by soaking the dried root in alcohol for several weeks, straining, and then using the tincture as a digestive aid.
- Dosage: Typically, a few drops of the tincture can be taken in water before meals to stimulate digestion.

Safety and Considerations:

Allergic Reactions: As with any herb, some people may experience allergic reactions to chicory, especially those who are sensitive to other members of the Asteraceae family, such as ragweed and daisies.

Pregnancy and Breastfeeding: Chicory is generally considered safe in food amounts, but due to its effects on menstruation and the gastrointestinal system, it should be used cautiously or avoided in medicinal amounts during pregnancy.

Interaction with Medications: Chicory may interact with certain medications due to its high inulin content, especially those involving the liver. If you are on medication, you should speak with your doctor.

Buchu, Agathosma botulina

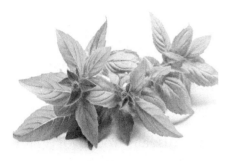

Composition:

- **Primary Components:** Contains volatile oils, including diosphenol (buchu camphor), which has antiseptic properties, as well as flavonoids and other phenolic compounds that contribute to its health benefits.
- **Other Phytochemicals:** Buchu also contains mucilages, which are thought to help soothe and coat the urinary tract during infections.

Buchu is a well-known remedy from South Africa, traditionally used by the Khoisan people. It's known for boosting energy, acting as a diuretic, and easing tummy troubles due to its strong scent. It's also a hit in Western herbal medicine as a natural urinary cleanser and diuretic, especially for fighting off bladder infections like cystitis. This herb, with its unique smell and flavor that's a bit like black currant with hints of rosemary and peppermint, thrives in South Africa's hillsides and is also grown in some South American regions. Buchu loves the sun and needs to be planted in soil that doesn't hold water. Its leaves are picked during the blooming or fruiting season in summer.

Uses

1. As a traditional South African remedy, buchu is taken to perk you up and help with water retention. Its strong aroma also helps with gas and bloating.

2. In today's Western herbal practices, buchu is still the go-to for urinary issues, much like it was back in the 19th century. It's often mixed with other herbs, such as cornsilk and juniper, to tackle urinary tract infections and can help keep recurring bladder or urethra inflammation at bay. It's also used for prostate and bladder irritations, usually paired with herbs like uva-ursi and cornsilk. The compound diosphenol in buchu may be what gives it its diuretic and antiseptic powers.

3. Buchu can be brewed into an infusion or made into a tincture for issues like cystitis and urethritis, particularly when they're connected to an underlying Candida problem, like yeast infections. The infusion is generally preferred when infections flare up suddenly. It's also used for vaginal issues like leukorrhea and sometimes yeast infections. However, because buchu can stimulate the uterus and contains pulegone – a compound that can induce abortion and menstrual flow – it's not safe for pregnant women.

Preparation:

1. Buchu Tea:

- Simple Preparation: Steep 1-2 teaspoons of dried buchu leaves in boiling water for about 10 minutes. Drink the tea after straining the leaves.
- Usage: Buchu tea is traditionally used for urinary tract health, and it's recommended to drink it 1-2 times a day when experiencing urinary issues.

2. Tincture:

- Alcohol Extraction: Soak dried buchu leaves in alcohol (usually vodka or grain alcohol) to create a tincture. This process extracts the active compounds effectively.
- Dosage: Tinctures are typically taken in small doses (a few drops in water), used to manage symptoms of UTIs and to promote kidney health.

3. Essential Oil:

- Extraction: Buchu essential oil is extracted from the leaves using steam distillation. It concentrates the plant's active chemicals.
- Topical Use: Dilute buchu essential oil with a carrier oil (like coconut oil) before applying to the skin, particularly for joint or muscle pain. It should not be applied undiluted due to its potency.

Safety and Considerations:

Pregnancy and Breastfeeding: Buchu is not recommended during pregnancy or breastfeeding due to potential risks, including stimulating the uterus.

Kidney Disease: Although used for kidney health, buchu should be used with caution in people with serious kidney diseases due to its potent diuretic properties.

Medication Interactions: Given its effects on the body's fluid balance, buchu may interact with diuretic medications and other treatments that affect blood pressure and kidney function.

Allergic Reactions: As with any herbal product, allergic reactions are possible, especially if you are sensitive to other plants in the Rutaceae family.

Chives, Allium schoenoprasum

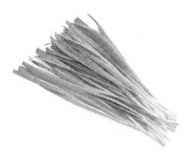

Composition:

• Primary Components: Chives are rich in vitamins A and C, which are important for immune function and skin health, respectively. They also contain vitamin K, which is essential for bone health and blood clotting.

• Other Phytochemicals: Contains allicin, which is converted from the precursor alliin when the plant is cut or crushed. Allicin has antimicrobial properties and may help lower blood pressure.

Allium schoenoprasum, commonly known as chives, is part of the Amaryllidaceae family, which also includes garlic, shallots, and leeks. These flavorful plants are a favorite in residential gardens and can also be found growing wild in various regions. They have a broad presence in North America, Europe, and Asia and are primarily used for culinary purposes. Chives are bulbous plants that reach heights between 12 to 20 inches (30 cm to 50 cm). Their slender bulbs measure roughly an inch (2.5 cm) in length and about half an inch (1.25 cm) in diameter, forming tightly packed clusters at the root. The stems are cylindrical, hollow, and can grow up to 20 inches (50 cm) in length, with a diameter of about an inch. They are more tender before the flowers bloom. Unlike the flat leaves of garlic chives (Allium tuberosum), chive leaves are grass-like, shorter than the stems, round in cross-section, and hollow.

In the southern regions, chives typically bloom from April to May, while in the north, they flower in June. The blossoms are generally a soft purple hue and appear in a compact bunch of 10 to 30 flowers, each cluster spanning ½ to 1 inch (1.25 cm to 2.5 cm) across. Before the flowers open, they are enclosed by a thin, papery covering. The fruit of the chive plant is a trifoliate capsule, and the seeds ripen during the summer.

Uses:

1. Chives are packed with sulfide compounds and agents that fight against bacteria and fungi, which can help soothe digestive issues and calm an upset stomach. They're also known to kickstart your appetite.

2. Similar to other members of the onion family, chives boast allicin, which is great for reducing harmful cholesterol levels. This contributes to a healthier circulatory system and heart. Eating chives regularly can help prevent the buildup of arterial deposits, ease blood vessel tension, lower high blood pressure, and reduce the risk of heart complications.

3. Rich in a variety of vitamins and minerals, including vitamin C, chives are fantastic for bolstering the immune system and encouraging the production of protective white blood cells.

4. With their gentle anti-inflammatory qualities, chives are a beneficial addition to meals, especially for those dealing with inflammatory conditions like arthritis, autoimmune diseases, and inflammatory skin issues.

Preparation:

1. Fresh Chives:

- Harvesting and Storage: Cut fresh chives with scissors about 2 inches above the ground to promote regrowth. Store fresh chives in the refrigerator wrapped lightly in a damp paper towel and placed inside a plastic bag.
- Using Fresh Chives: Snip fresh chives with scissors directly over dishes to preserve their flavor and nutritional content. They are best added towards the end of cooking to maintain their delicate flavor.

2. Dried Chives:

- Drying Process: To dry chives, tie them in small bundles and hang them in a dry, well-ventilated area away from direct sunlight. After they've dried, put them somewhere airtight and dark.
- Use of Dried Chives: Dried chives can be rehydrated in a little water and used as a substitute for fresh chives, although the flavor will be milder.

3. Chive Butter:

- Making Flavored Butter: Mix finely chopped chives into softened butter to make chive butter. This can be used as a spread or to finish dishes like steaks, fish, or potatoes.
- Storage: Chive butter can be rolled into logs and wrapped in wax paper. For extended storage, place in the freezer or refrigerate.

4. Chive Oil:

- Infusion: Infuse mild olive oil or vegetable oil with chopped chives for a few weeks in a cool, dark place, then strain.
- Usage: Use chive oil as a dressing for salads or drizzled over cooked dishes to add a subtle onion-like flavor.

Safety and Considerations:

Allergies: Being part of the Allium family, chives may cause an allergic reaction in people sensitive to onions, garlic, and other similar plants.

Nutrient Stability: Vitamin C and some other sensitive phytochemicals in chives can be degraded by prolonged cooking; thus, adding chives at the end of cooking or using them raw helps preserve their nutritional value.

Bupleurum, B. scorzoneraefolium

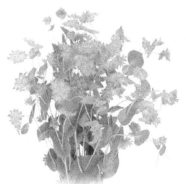

Composition:

• Primary Components: Contains a group of saponins known as saikosaponins, which have anti-inflammatory, antipyretic, and liver-protecting effects.
• Other Phytochemicals: Also includes flavonoids, essential oils, and polysaccharides, contributing to its overall health benefits.

Bupleurum, a plant first recorded in writings dating back to the 1st century BCE, is celebrated in Chinese herbal medicine for creating harmony within the body by balancing various organs and internal energies. It's known for its invigorating effects, particularly on the digestive system and liver, and for its ability to increase blood circulation to the skin's surface. Japanese studies have recently confirmed its liver-protecting benefits, aligning with its historical use. This herb thrives in China, especially in the central and eastern regions, and it can also be found across Asia and Europe. Bupleurum is grown from seeds in the spring or from root cuttings in the fall, and it prefers sunny spots with soil that drains well. Harvesting of the root typically happens in spring and fall.

Uses

1. In China, bupleurum has been a go-to liver enhancer for more than two millennia. It's thought to boost liver qi and support the spleen and stomach. When the liver and spleen are out of sync, resulting in digestive woes like stomachaches, bloating, queasiness, and poor digestion, bupleurum is the herb of choice.

2. Similar to milk thistle and licorice from the Glycyrrhiza family, bupleurum is a top pick for tackling liver issues, thanks to its anti-inflammatory properties that aid in managing liver conditions.

3. For those battling fevers, the flu, or colds, particularly with symptoms like a bitter taste, moodiness, and either throwing up with stomach pain or feeling dizzy and lightheaded, bupleurum is a popular remedy in China.

4. The synergy between traditional bupleurum uses and scientific findings is so strong that many Japanese doctors, even those trained in Western medicine, prescribe bupleurum root extracts to patients with liver ailments.

5. Bupleurum can also be helpful in treating hemorrhoids and pelvic issues, such as a dropped uterus.

Preparation:

1. Decoction:

- Traditional Preparation: Bupleurum roots are typically used to make a decoction. To do this, add about 3-9 grams of the dried root to boiling water, simmer for 30 minutes to several hours depending on the desired strength.
- Combination: It is often combined with other herbs such as ginseng, ginger, and licorice in traditional Chinese medicine formulas to balance its potent effects and target specific conditions.

2. Tincture:

- Alcohol Extraction: The roots can also be used to make a tincture by soaking them in alcohol for several weeks. This method extracts the active compounds effectively and is used for easier dosing and absorption.
- Usage: Typically, tinctures are taken in small amounts (a few drops to a teaspoon) diluted in water, one to three times a day.

3. Powder:

- Ground Root: The dried root can be ground into a powder and used to make capsules or mixed into liquids.
- Dosage: This form is convenient for controlling dosage and combining with other powdered herbs.

Safety and Considerations:

Side Effects: Bupleurum can cause side effects such as increased bowel movements, flatulence, and drowsiness. High doses can lead to more severe reactions, including nausea and vomiting.

Pregnancy and Breastfeeding: It is generally advised to avoid Bupleurum during pregnancy and breastfeeding due to its strong effects and lack of safety data.

Interactions with Medications: Due to its effects on the liver and immune system, Bupleurum may interact with medications that are metabolized by the liver or that affect the immune system. It's important to consult with a healthcare provider if you are on any such medications.

Comfrey, Symphytum officinale

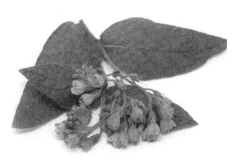

Composition:

- **Primary Components:** Contains allantoin, a compound that promotes cell growth and repair, making it effective for skin and tissue healing.
- **Other Phytochemicals:** Comfrey also includes rosmarinic acid, which has anti-inflammatory properties, and mucilage, which is soothing to the skin. However, the presence of pyrrolizidine alkaloids raises concerns about liver toxicity if ingested.

Comfrey belongs to the borage family and thrives like a wild plant in many places. It's a breeze to grow in your backyard and is also known by names like knit bone, boneset, and slippery root. This hardy perennial sports long, lance-shaped leaves that can stretch from 12 to 18 inches. It sprouts hairy leaves from a central crown atop short stems, standing tall at 2 to 5 feet and spreading out to over 3 feet wide. You can start it from cuttings, and it won't take over your garden. Its flowers start off blue or purple, then turn pink over time. Comfrey's thick roots are covered in a slender black outer layer.

Uses

1. Comfrey is a top-notch healer for skin and wounds, slashing the risk of infection and scarring thanks to its bacteria-fighting powers. It's full of a substance called allantoin that speeds up cell repair. Plus, it's a champ at easing inflammation and pain in joints and muscles. Drinking comfrey tea can help with stomach troubles, heavy periods, blood in urine, respiratory issues, cancer, and heart pain. But, heads up—be cautious with drinking it (more on that in a bit). It's also good as a mouth rinse for gum issues or a sore throat.

2. Got a sprain, muscle bruise, joint injury, or even a broken bone? Comfrey to the rescue! It can help you heal faster, get moving sooner, and take the edge off the pain and swelling. Slather on some comfrey salve or slap on a poultice made from the root up to four times daily. Just ensure any broken bones are properly set before you go the comfrey route.

3. For minor skin boo-boos like rashes, eczema, burns, and cuts, comfrey is your go-to. It works wonders, especially the root, but leaves are good too. Apply a comfrey salve thrice a day or use a poultice for quick healing. Washing the area with Comfrey Tea or a root decoction is great for skin irritations like acne or psoriasis. But, steer clear of using it on deep or puncture wounds—it's so good at healing, it might trap infections inside. And a word of caution: it could be risky for your liver or during pregnancy, so if you've got liver issues or are expecting, it's best to avoid it.

4. If you're dealing with knee or joint pain from osteoarthritis, an external application of comfrey salve can provide some much-needed relief.

Preparation:

1. Topical Applications:

- Comfrey Salve: You can make a comfrey salve by infusing the leaves or roots in a carrier oil (like olive or coconut oil) over low heat for several hours, then mixing with beeswax until thickened. This salve can be applied externally to help heal cuts, bruises, and sprains.
- Comfrey Poultice: Crush fresh comfrey leaves to make a poultice and apply it directly to the affected area to reduce swelling and pain in cases of sprains or bone injuries.

2. Comfrey Tea for External Use:

- Simple Preparation: Steep dried comfrey leaves or root in boiling water for 10-15 minutes, then allow cooling. Use this tea as a compress or wash for skin irritations and injuries.
- Note: It is recommended to use comfrey tea externally only, due to the risk of liver damage from internal consumption.

Safety and Considerations:

Toxicity Concerns: Comfrey contains pyrrolizidine alkaloids, which are hepatotoxic and potentially carcinogenic if ingested. Therefore, it should not be taken internally or used on open wounds that might allow PAs to enter the bloodstream.

Regulatory Restrictions: In many countries, the sale of comfrey products is regulated, especially those intended for internal use.

Duration of Use: Even for external use, it is advised not to use comfrey for extended periods (not more than 10 consecutive days) due to potential systemic absorption of PAs.

Pregnancy and Breastfeeding: Avoid using comfrey during pregnancy and breastfeeding due to the lack of safety data and potential for toxicity.

Common Flax, Linum usitatissimum

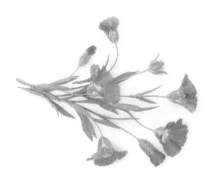

Composition:

- **Primary Components:** Flaxseeds are rich in alpha-linolenic acid (ALA), a type of omega-3 fatty acid. They also contain high levels of lignans, which have antioxidant properties and may help balance hormones.
- **Other Phytochemicals:** Flaxseeds are a great source of soluble and insoluble dietary fibers and contain vitamins like vitamin B1 and minerals such as magnesium.

Also referred to as Flaxseed, this versatile plant is sought after for its medicinal properties, oil extraction, and textile production. It's a popular dietary addition for its health benefits and belongs to the Linaceae, or Flax, family. Typically an annual plant, Common Flax seldom grows in the wild but is easy to cultivate or find as a crop. When fully grown, it reaches a height of 3 to 4 feet. At the top of its branching stems, it sports a cluster of blue-purple flowers on stalks, each flower being about ¾ to 1 inch across with five ovate petals, encircled by five upright, blue-tipped stamens and a green center. The sepals are lance-shaped. Flax's simple green leaves are alternate, straight, and without stalks, ranging from 1/2 to 1 1/2 inches in length, with smooth edges. The plant typically has straight, unbranched stems with multiple smooth, round stems at its base. Its fruit is a round, dry capsule with five lobes, measuring between 1/4 and 1/2 inch in diameter.

Uses:

1. Flaxseed is loaded with dietary fiber, protein, omega-3s, and other valuable nutrients. You can personally grind flax and chia seeds every day for your well-being, as fresh seeds are preferable since their oil can spoil quickly.

2. Regular consumption of ground flaxseeds can help reduce cholesterol and LDL levels.

3. Rich in omega-3 fatty acids, alpha-linolenic acid (ALA), and lignans, flaxseeds support the immune system, reduce inflammation, offer neuroprotection, act as antioxidants, and influence hormones in autoimmune diseases.

4. Flaxseed oil can alleviate respiratory issues, including ARDS. Its anti-inflammatory properties can soothe coughs, sore throats, and congestion.

5. If you're dealing with constipation, two teaspoons of ground flaxseed with a large glass of water each morning could be beneficial.

6. Flaxseed contains lignans, which are phytoestrogens that can help balance female hormones, particularly after menopause, easing symptoms.

7. As a supportive treatment and preventive measure, both flaxseed and its oil may contribute to the management of breast and prostate cancers, potentially lowering PSA levels and reducing risks. Always discuss with your cancer specialist before trying new treatments.

Preparation:

1. Whole Flaxseeds:

- Basic Use: You can add whole flaxseeds directly to your diet by sprinkling them over salads, cereals, and yogurt. However, whole seeds are often not fully digested, which means you might not get all the nutrients.

2. Ground Flaxseed:

- Grinding: To make the nutrients more bioavailable, grind flaxseeds in a coffee grinder or food processor. Ground flaxseed can be added to smoothies, baked goods, and more.
- Storage: Keep ground flaxseed in an airtight container in the refrigerator to prevent it from going rancid quickly due to its high fat content.

3. Flaxseed Oil:

- Extraction: Flaxseed oil is extracted from the seeds and should be purchased cold-pressed and stored in the refrigerator to maintain its nutritional quality.
- Usage: Use flaxseed oil as a dressing for salads or drizzle over cooked dishes; it should not be used for high-temperature cooking as it oxidizes easily.

4. Flaxseed Tea:

- Simple Tea Preparation: Boil one tablespoon of ground flaxseed in a cup of water for about 8-10 minutes, strain, and drink.
- Benefits: Flaxseed tea is used for soothing the digestive tract and relieving constipation due to its mucilaginous fiber content.

Safety and Considerations:

Digestive Effects: Consuming large amounts of flaxseed can lead to gastrointestinal discomfort, bloating, and laxative effects. Increase gradually after starting with smaller quantities.

Pregnancy and Breastfeeding: Flaxseeds are generally considered safe during pregnancy and breastfeeding, but it is best to consume them in moderation.

Blood Thinning Properties: Flaxseeds may have a blood-thinning effect due to their high omega-3 content. If you are taking blood-thinning medications (like warfarin), consult your healthcare provider before adding significant amounts of flaxseed to your diet.

Cayenne, Capsicum annuum & C. frutescens

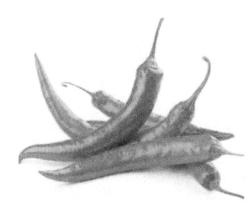

Composition:

- **Primary Components:** Contains capsaicin, which is the compound responsible for the chili's heat. Capsaicin is known for its pain-relief properties and effects on metabolism.
- **Other Phytochemicals:** Cayenne peppers are also rich in vitamins A, B6, C, and E, as well as potassium and manganese.

Cayenne pepper, which hails from the warm regions of the Americas, found its way to Europe around the 1500s. It's famous in the kitchen for its fiery flavor, and it's no shock that it doubles as a potent herbal booster. It gets the blood pumping and aids digestion, offering relief for everything from joint pain and frost-nipped toes to stomach cramps and the runs. This spicy plant calls the tropical Americas its home and is now a hot crop across the globe, thriving under the sun in places like Africa and India. Planted in the early throes of spring, cayenne loves the steamy weather. Come summertime, its fruits are plucked and left to dry out of the sun's glare.

Uses:

1. Feeling chilly in your fingers and toes? Cayenne's like a cozy blanket for your blood vessels, getting that warm blood where it needs to go.

2. The ancient Mayans were onto something—they used cayenne to fight off nasty bugs. Turns out, cayenne's got some serious germ-fighting chops. Sprinkle it in your meals, and you might just dodge a tummy trouble or two. Herbalists are big fans, using it to soothe upset stomachs and more severe tummy troubles.

3. Got a case of the aches? Rub a bit of cayenne on your skin. It's like a gentle fire that eases pain and gets the blood flowing, especially in those stiff, "cold" joints. It's also a champ for those pesky, non-broken chilblains.

4. If you're feeling bloated or battling bellyaches, cayenne's your go-to. It kicks your digestive juices into gear and can be a little helper for a heart that's not quite up to speed. A smidge in your gargle can soothe a scratchy throat, and it's even got a knack for calming sudden diarrhea.

Preparation:

1. Dried and Ground:

- Preparation: Cayenne peppers are often dried and ground into a fine powder. This powder can be used as a spice in cooking or as a supplement in capsule form.
- Usage: Add ground cayenne pepper to dishes for heat and flavor or take capsules as directed for dietary supplementation.

2. Cayenne Tincture:

- Alcohol Extraction: Soak dried cayenne pepper in alcohol to create a tincture. This method concentrates the active ingredients and can be used medicinally.
- Dosage: Use a few drops of the tincture in water or apply topically, diluted with a carrier oil, for pain relief.

3. Cayenne Oil or Salve:

- Infusion: Infuse cayenne into a carrier oil (like olive or coconut oil) for several weeks. Strain out the solids. The resulting cayenne oil can be used topically to relieve joint and muscle pain.
- Salve: Combine the infused oil with beeswax to make a salve that can be applied to painful areas.

Safety and Considerations:

Gastrointestinal Irritation: While cayenne can aid in digestion, it can also irritate the gastrointestinal tract, especially in those who are not accustomed to spicy foods or who have a gastrointestinal disorder.

Topical Use Sensitivity: When used topically, cayenne can cause irritation, burning sensations, and even dermatitis. Always use diluted with a carrier oil and test on a small area first.

Pregnancy and Breastfeeding: Generally, cayenne is safe in food amounts during pregnancy and breastfeeding but should be used cautiously in medicinal amounts due to its potent effects.

Interactions: Cayenne might interact with certain medications, including ACE inhibitors and stomach acid reducers. It's also a blood thinner, so it should be used with caution if you are taking blood-thinning medications.

Couch Grass, Agropyron repens

Composition:

- **Primary Components:** Couch grass contains mucilage, which gives it soothing properties, and saponins, which contribute to its diuretic effects. It also contains small amounts of silica, potassium, and other minerals.
- **Other Phytochemicals:** Couch grass also contains polysaccharides and sterols, which may contribute to its medicinal properties.

Couch Grass, also referred to as quackgrass, dog grass, witchgrass, or twitch grass, is often dismissed as a pesky weed, yet it boasts an array of health benefits that shouldn't be overlooked. This member of the Poaceae family can tower up to 3 feet tall and is recognized by its creeping, elongated roots and slim leaves. From late June to August, it flourishes, producing flower spikes with small, oval spikelets. Despite its invasive tendencies, particularly in agricultural settings, couch grass thrives in loose, sandy soils but struggles in compacted earth.

Uses

1. Brew up a couch grass decoction to tackle gout.

2. Thanks to its anti-inflammatory and diuretic effects, plus its support for urinary and gallbladder health, couch grass is a solid pick for managing jaundice, helping the body detoxify and recover.

3. For urinary tract issues like inflammation, infections, or painful urination due to bladder or urethra spasms, couch grass can be soothing. It acts as a diuretic, boosting urine flow, breaking down kidney stones, and combating cystitis and gallbladder conditions. Combine it with Usnea and bearberry for a potent urinary tract infection remedy.

4. The combined diuretic, anti-inflammatory, and pain-relieving properties make couch grass a useful ally against rheumatoid arthritis.

Preparation:

1. Couch Grass Tea:

- Simple Preparation: Add 1-2 teaspoons of dried couch grass rhizome (underground stem) to a cup of boiling water. Allow it to steep for 10-15 minutes, then strain and drink.

- Usage: Couch grass tea is typically consumed 1-3 times per day as a diuretic to help increase urine flow and promote urinary tract health.

2. Tincture:

- Alcohol Extraction: Couch grass can also be prepared as a tincture by soaking the dried rhizome in alcohol for several weeks, then straining. The tincture can be taken in small doses diluted in water.
- Dosage: Follow the instructions on the tincture bottle or consult with a herbalist for appropriate dosing.

Safety and Considerations:

Allergic Reactions: Some individuals may experience allergic reactions to couch grass, particularly those who are sensitive to grass pollens.

Pregnancy and Breastfeeding: While couch grass is generally considered safe, pregnant and breastfeeding women should consult a healthcare provider before using it as a herbal remedy.

Interactions: Couch grass may interact with certain medications, particularly diuretics and medications that affect electrolyte balance. It's important to consult with a healthcare provider before using couch grass if you are on medication.

Senna, Senna alexandrina

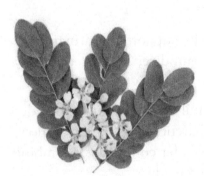

Composition:

- Primary Components: Senna contains anthraquinone glycosides, particularly sennosides A and B, which are responsible for its laxative effects. These compounds stimulate the muscles in the intestines, promoting bowel movements.
- Other Phytochemicals: Senna also contains flavonoids, which have antioxidant properties.

Moving on to senna, this well-known herbal remedy is a go-to for many, especially since it's commonly used in modern medicine as a potent laxative. Originating from tropical Africa, senna thrives in sunny conditions and is harvested for its leaves and ripe pods. Despite its somewhat bitter and off-putting taste, it's often blended with other herbs to make it more palatable.

Uses

1. Senna is a classic choice for relieving constipation, particularly when a soft stool is necessary, like with anal fissures. It's effective as a short-term laxative but shouldn't be used for extended periods (no more than 10 days) to prevent weakening the muscles of the large intestine.

2. As a powerful laxative, senna can sometimes cause cramping or colic, so it's usually taken with carminative herbs that help relax the intestines and alleviate discomfort.

Preparation:

1. Senna Tea:

- Simple Preparation: Add 1-2 teaspoons of dried senna leaves or crushed senna pods to a cup of boiling water. After letting it steep for 5 - 10 minutes, strain and enjoy.
- Usage: Senna tea is typically consumed at bedtime to produce a bowel movement the following morning. Start with a low dose and adjust as needed to avoid discomfort.

2. Senna Capsules or Tablets:

- Commercial Preparation: Senna is also available in capsule or tablet form, often in combination with other herbal laxatives. Follow the dosage instructions on the product label or as directed by a healthcare provider.

3. Senna Tincture:

- Extraction: Senna can be prepared as a tincture by soaking the dried leaves or pods in alcohol for several weeks, then straining. The tincture can be taken in small doses diluted in water.
- Dosage: Follow the instructions on the tincture bottle or consult with a healthcare provider for appropriate dosing.

Safety and Considerations:

Short-Term Use: Senna is safe for short-term use to relieve occasional constipation. However, long-term or frequent use can lead to dependence and other complications, such as electrolyte imbalance and dehydration.

Pregnancy and Breastfeeding: Pregnant and breastfeeding women should avoid using senna, as it may stimulate uterine contractions and pass into breast milk, potentially causing diarrhea in infants.

Side Effects: Side effects of senna may include abdominal cramps, diarrhea, nausea, and electrolyte imbalances. It should be used with caution in individuals with gastrointestinal disorders or electrolyte abnormalities.

Dandelion, Taraxacum officinale

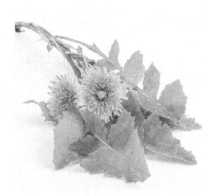

Composition:

• **Primary Components:** Dandelion contains various bioactive compounds, including sesquiterpene lactones, phenolic compounds, flavonoids, and vitamins (such as vitamin A, C, and K).

• **Other Phytochemicals:** It also contains inulin, a type of soluble fiber that acts as a prebiotic, supporting the growth of beneficial gut bacteria.

Kids absolutely love the chance to scatter dandelion seeds into the breeze. This delightful plant, often dismissed as a pesky weed, pops up in the most unexpected places like the crevices of sidewalks and the wild, unkempt areas of roadsides and yards. But be careful— there are a few plants that look just like it, so make sure you've got the right one before you go picking it. Dandelions, part of the Aster/Daisy family, are hardy little things that originally hail from North America. They've got this deep-reaching taproot and can grow about a foot tall. They bloom with these bright yellow flowers made up of tiny florets from April through June. The leaves have this unique, jagged look, kind of like a lion's teeth, which is actually how they got their name.

Uses

1. You can use the whole plant for health benefits. The roots are super bitter but great for your gut and liver, while the leaves can help you get rid of extra water in your body. Dandelions are like a health boost for your whole system, packed with vitamins, minerals, and antioxidants. Personally, I'm a fan of dandelion tea or a tincture for taking it internally.

2. Dandelions are also rich in iron and other nutrients. Iron's crucial for your blood, keeping those red blood cells in tip-top shape. Eating dandelion greens or using them in other ways can help keep your iron levels up.

3. If you're looking to drop your blood pressure, dandelion juice is your friend because it helps your body get rid of extra salt. Plus, it can improve your cholesterol balance by increasing the good stuff.

4. Boosting your immune system is another dandelion perk. It's like your body's personal bouncer, keeping those nasty bugs and fungi at bay.

5. Got a scrape or a skin issue? Dandelion juice to the rescue! It speeds up healing and fights off the germs that cause infections. The sap, or the "milk" from the stem, works wonders on itches, ringworm, eczema, warts, and even corns. Just dab it on! You can also use dandelion

tea as a skin wash. And if acne's a problem, dandelion's got your back—it helps prevent breakouts and reduces scarring. Just a heads-up, though—some folks might be allergic, so do a patch test first.

6. For your bones, dandelions are like a shield against osteoporosis and arthritis, thanks to the calcium and vitamin K they contain. They help keep your bones strong and sturdy.

7. And let's not forget about inflammation. Dandelions are full of stuff that helps reduce swelling and pain. This is super important because inflammation can lead to all sorts of problems, like arthritis. There's this compound in dandelion roots, taraxasterol, that's showing some real potential for helping with osteoarthritis.

Preparation:

1. Dandelion Tea:

- Simple Preparation: Steep dried dandelion roots or leaves in boiling water for about 5-10 minutes. Strain and drink.
- Usage: Dandelion tea can be consumed daily to support liver health, aid digestion, and promote detoxification. It can also be combined with other herbs for enhanced effects.

2. Dandelion Tincture:

- Alcohol Extraction: Dandelion roots or leaves can be soaked in alcohol to create a tincture. This method concentrates the active ingredients and can be used medicinally.
- Dosage: Follow the instructions on the tincture bottle or as directed by a healthcare provider.

3. Dandelion Greens:

- Culinary Use: Dandelion greens can be eaten raw in salads or cooked like spinach. They have a slightly bitter taste and are rich in nutrients, including vitamins A, C, and K.

4. Dandelion Root Coffee:

- Preparation: Roast dried dandelion roots until they are dark and fragrant, then grind them to a fine powder. Brew the ground roots as you would coffee.
- Usage: Dandelion root coffee is caffeine-free and can be enjoyed as a coffee substitute, with potential benefits for liver health and digestion.

Safety and Considerations:

Allergic Reactions: Some individuals may be allergic to dandelion pollen or other parts of the plant. If you have allergies to plants in the Asteraceae family, use caution when consuming dandelion.

Interactions: Dandelion may interact with certain medications, particularly blood thinners and diuretics. Consult with a healthcare provider before using dandelion supplements if you are taking medication.

Pregnancy and Breastfeeding: While dandelion is generally considered safe when consumed in moderation as food, pregnant and breastfeeding women should avoid using dandelion supplements or medicinal doses without consulting a healthcare provider.

Gotu Kola, Hydrocotyle asiatica

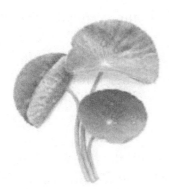

Composition:

• Primary Components: Gotu kola contains triterpenoid compounds, including asiaticoside, asiatic acid, and madecassic acid, which are believed to be responsible for its medicinal properties.

• Other Phytochemicals: It also contains flavonoids, phenolic compounds, and other antioxidants, which contribute to its overall health benefits.

Gotu kola, a time-honored remedy from Ayurvedic traditions, has found widespread use in Western cultures. This versatile herb is known for its skin-healing and digestive-aiding properties. In India, it's employed to combat various ailments, including leprosy, but it's primarily cherished for its ability to enhance nerve health and boost memory. It has a unique taste that's both bittersweet and slightly sharp, and it's even tossed into salads and cooked as a green in Indian cuisine. This plant calls India and the southern United States its home, thriving in warm, moist climates across parts of Australia, southern Africa, and South America, often along riverbanks and in swampy regions. While typically harvested in the wild, gotu kola can also be grown from seeds in the spring, with its above-ground parts collected year-round.

Uses

1. Gotu kola is renowned for its effectiveness in healing wounds and tackling skin issues. Ayurvedic practices utilize it to speed up recovery from skin ulcers and severe skin conditions, aiming to minimize scarring. Whether applied topically or ingested, it seems to stimulate tissue repair body-wide. It's also praised for enhancing peripheral blood flow and is taken to

fortify blood vessels, such as those affected by varicose veins. Many advocates believe in its power to stave off and alleviate arthritis and rheumatic discomfort.

2. In India and South Asia, the herb is celebrated as a "rejuvenator," known to improve focus and memory, especially among older adults. Western herbalists recognize it as an adaptogen, suggesting its long-term consumption for sustained brain health, aging gracefully, and easing stress. It's also believed to act as a digestive tonic.

Preparation:

1. Gotu Kola Tea:

- Simple Preparation: Add dried gotu kola leaves to boiling water and let steep for 5-10 minutes. Strain and drink.
- Usage: Gotu kola tea can be consumed daily to support overall health and well-being. It has a mild, slightly bitter taste.

2. Gotu Kola Tincture:

- Alcohol Extraction: Soak dried gotu kola leaves in alcohol to create a tincture. This method concentrates the active compounds and can be used medicinally.
- Dosage: Follow the instructions on the tincture bottle or as directed by a healthcare provider.

3. Gotu Kola Extract:

- Liquid or Capsules: Gotu kola extract is available in liquid form or as capsules. Follow the dosage instructions on the product label or as directed by a healthcare provider.

Safety and Considerations:

Pregnancy and Breastfeeding: Gotu kola is generally considered safe when consumed in moderate amounts during pregnancy and breastfeeding. However, high doses should be avoided, and it's best to consult a healthcare provider before use.

Allergic Reactions: Some individuals may be allergic to gotu kola, particularly if they are sensitive to plants in the Apiaceae family.

Interactions: Gotu kola may interact with certain medications, including blood thinners and medications that affect liver function. Consult with a healthcare provider before using gotu kola supplements if you are taking medication.

Dill, Anethum graveolens

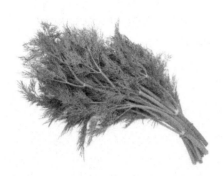

Composition:

- **Primary Components:** Dill contains essential oils, including carvone and limonene, which contribute to its flavor and aroma. It also contains flavonoids, phenolic compounds, and vitamins (such as vitamin C and vitamin A).
- **Nutritional Content:** Dill is low in calories but rich in antioxidants, vitamins, and minerals. It provides small amounts of fiber, calcium, iron, magnesium, and potassium.

Dill is a popular herb known for its aromatic qualities and is widely grown in herb gardens throughout the nation. It belongs to the Apiaceae or Umbelliferae family, which includes celery and carrots. The plant stands about 30 inches tall with a thin, hollow stem that stands upright and sports delicate, feathery foliage. The leaves, which resemble those of fennel, range from 4 to 8 inches in length and are finely segmented, giving them a gentle look. As the weather heats up, clusters of small yellow or white blossoms emerge, forming umbrellas between 3/4 and 3 1/2 inches across. The seeds are tiny, no more than 1/5 inch long, and feature a grooved texture.

Uses:

1. A dill water concoction is great for soothing colicky infants. It eases stomach discomfort and calms the little ones down. It's a go-to remedy for colic because it's easy to get, works well, and is recognized as safe for kids.

2. If you're dealing with cramps or muscle spasms, including those in the gut, a dill leaf brew can offer quick relief. It eases the pain of spasms without addressing the root cause. You can use it for immediate comfort while you figure out what's actually wrong. A brew made from dill seeds or a dill extract can be helpful, too.

3. To freshen your breath temporarily, just chew on some dill leaves or seeds. But if you want a lasting solution, chewing seeds regularly can tackle the underlying issues behind bad breath.

4. Dill brew can also be a boon for breastfeeding moms, helping to increase milk production. Plus, it has a calming effect on both mother and baby.

5. To combat gas, try having a dill seed brew before meals.

Preparation:

1. Fresh Dill:

- Harvesting: Fresh dill leaves can be harvested from the plant as needed. Simply snip off the desired amount with scissors or a knife.
- Usage: Fresh dill leaves are commonly used as a garnish for dishes, particularly in salads, soups, seafood, and sauces.

2. Dried Dill:

- Drying Process: Dill leaves can be dried by hanging them upside down in a well-ventilated area until they are completely dry. For later usage, they can be kept dry in an airtight container.
- Usage: Dried dill can be used in place of fresh dill in recipes that require longer cooking times, such as stews and casseroles.

3. Dill Seeds:

- Harvesting: Dill seeds are the mature fruits of the dill plant and can be harvested once they have turned brown and dry.
- Usage: Dill seeds are often used as a spice in pickling brines, marinades, and spice blends. They have a slightly stronger flavor than dill leaves and add a unique aroma to dishes.

Safety and Considerations:

Allergic Reactions: Some individuals may be allergic to dill or other members of the Apiaceae family, such as celery, parsley, and fennel. Use caution if you have known allergies to these plants.

Pregnancy and Breastfeeding: Dill is generally considered safe when consumed in moderate amounts as a food ingredient. However, medicinal doses or supplements should be avoided during pregnancy and breastfeeding.

Medication Interactions: Dill may interact with certain medications, particularly blood thinners and medications that affect blood sugar levels. Consult with a healthcare provider if you are taking medication and considering dill supplements.

Chrysanthemum, Chrysanthemum x morifolium

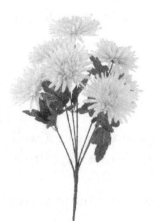

Composition:

• **Primary Components:** Chrysanthemum flowers contain various bioactive compounds, including flavonoids (such as luteolin and apigenin), phenolic acids, and essential oils.

• **Nutritional Content:** While not commonly consumed for their nutritional content, chrysanthemum flowers contain small amounts of vitamins and minerals.

Chrysanthemum isn't just a pretty face! While it's known for its beauty, in China, it's also a go-to herb for health. People there sip it as a soothing tea. It's got a reputation for sharpening sight and calming irritated eyes, easing head pains, and fighting off those pesky colds and sniffles. Plus, studies say it's a champ at managing high blood pressure. This flower is a true local, originating from China, where it's now mostly farm-grown. It's reproduced from cuttings when the weather warms up. Come fall, when the blooms are at their peak, they're picked and sun-dried, which might take a while.

Uses

1. For ages, the Chinese have turned to chrysanthemum as a trusty herbal fix and a delightful drink, dating back to the 1st century CE in the Divine Husbandman's Classic.

2. Tired, sore eyes from too much screen time or reading? The Chinese have a trick: they use the warmed-up flowers as a compress to give their eyes a break. Drinking the tea is also a popular way to boost eye health.

3. Feeling feverish or under the weather? Chrysanthemum tea to the rescue! It helps bring down fevers, relieves stress headaches, moistens a parched mouth or throat, and even freshens your breath.

4. Got skin troubles? The fresh leaves can be mashed into a natural antiseptic mash for pesky skin issues like acne or boils.

5. If high blood pressure has you dealing with dizziness, headaches, or ringing in the ears, chrysanthemum might just be what you need to feel better.

Preparation:

1. Chrysanthemum Tea:

- Simple Preparation: Add dried chrysanthemum flowers to boiling water and let steep for 5-10 minutes. Strain and drink.
- Usage: Chrysanthemum tea is commonly consumed for its refreshing flavor and potential health benefits. It tastes good either hot or cold and is frequently sweetened with sugar or honey.

2. Chrysanthemum Tincture:

- Alcohol Extraction: Chrysanthemum flowers can be soaked in alcohol to create a tincture. This method concentrates the active compounds and can be used medicinally.
- Dosage: Follow the instructions on the tincture bottle or as directed by a healthcare provider.

3. Culinary Use:

- Edible Flowers: Chrysanthemum flowers can be used as a decorative garnish for salads, soups, desserts, and beverages. They add a pop of color and a subtle floral flavor to dishes.

Safety and Considerations:

Allergic Reactions: Some individuals may be allergic to chrysanthemum flowers, particularly those who are sensitive to plants in the Asteraceae family.

Pregnancy and Breastfeeding: While chrysanthemum tea is generally considered safe when consumed in moderate amounts, pregnant and breastfeeding women should avoid excessive consumption.

Medication Interactions: Chrysanthemum may interact with certain medications, particularly blood thinners and medications that affect blood sugar levels. Consult with a healthcare provider if you are taking medication and considering chrysanthemum supplements.

Dock, Rumex crispus

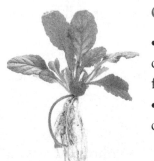

Composition:

• 	Primary Components: Dock contains various bioactive compounds, including anthraquinones (such as emodin), tannins, flavonoids, and vitamins (such as vitamin C).

• 	Nutritional Content: Dock leaves are rich in vitamins A and C, calcium, iron, and other minerals.

The Rumex genus, part of the Polygonaceae or Buckwheat family, encompasses over 200 species, including the well-known Rumex crispus, renowned for its healing properties. Similarly, the broad-leaved dock, Rumex obtusifolius, shares comparable uses. Globally found, the Curly Dock, also known as yellow dock, sour dock, narrow-leaved dock, or curled dock, is a biennial herb. It features a rosette-like base from which flower stalks emerge, topped with clusters of large, leathery leaves that are wavy or curly at the edges and have a rough texture. These leaves can reach lengths of up to two feet but are typically only about three inches wide, with small veins that arc towards the edges before turning back towards the central vein. The size and appearance of leaves can vary higher up on the plant, and older leaves sometimes have a reddish hue along the central vein. The flower stalk stands around three feet tall, bearing clustered flowers and seeds in its second year. The tiny green flowers form dense heads, and the three-sided seeds are encased in a papery, heart-shaped wing-like sheath. Below ground, the plant is anchored by a long, forking yellow taproot that helps it regenerate year after year.

Uses

1. The root of the Curly Dock acts as a bitter tonic, particularly benefiting the gallbladder and liver by boosting bile production and aiding the body's detoxification processes. It's especially useful for conditions that require the body to be purified of toxins and is often paired with Greater Burdock to enhance the detox effect.

2. As a gentle and safe laxative, Curly Dock can help ease mild constipation. Interestingly, it can also either cause or alleviate diarrhea, depending on how much is used and other variables like when it was harvested and the soil it grew in.

3. This versatile plant also finds use in treating numerous skin issues due to its cleansing properties. Whether taken internally as a tonic or externally as a poultice, salve, or powder, the dried or crushed root can be applied to treat sores, wounds, or various skin conditions.

Preparation:

1. Dock Leaves:

- Harvesting: Young dock leaves can be harvested in spring and early summer before they become tough and bitter. Keep an eye out for fragile, brilliant green leaves.
- Usage: Dock leaves can be cooked and eaten like spinach or added to salads, soups, stews, and omelets. Their flavor is acidic and slightly sour.

2. Dock Root:

- Harvesting: Dock roots can be harvested in autumn when they are mature. Wash and scrub the roots thoroughly to remove dirt and debris.
- Preparation: Dock roots can be dried and powdered for use in herbal remedies. They can also be decocted or infused in hot water to make tea.
- Usage: Dock root tea is commonly consumed for its potential health benefits, particularly for digestive health and detoxification.

Safety and Considerations:

Oxalic Acid Content: Dock leaves contain oxalic acid, which can interfere with calcium absorption and may exacerbate kidney stone formation in susceptible individuals. Cooking can help reduce oxalic acid levels.

Allergic Reactions: Some individuals may be allergic to dock pollen or other parts of the plant. Use caution if you have known allergies to plants in the Polygonaceae family.

Pregnancy and Breastfeeding: While dock is generally considered safe when consumed in moderate amounts as food, pregnant and breastfeeding women should avoid excessive consumption and consult with a healthcare provider before using dock supplements or medicinal doses.

Black Cohosh, Actaea racemosa

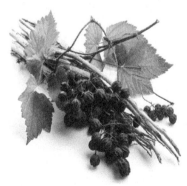

Composition:

- Primary Components: Black cohosh contains various bioactive compounds, including triterpene glycosides (such as actein and cimicifugoside), phenolic acids, and flavonoids (such as formononetin and kaempferol).
- Nutritional Content: Black cohosh is not commonly consumed for its nutritional content but contains small amounts of vitamins and minerals.

Black cohosh, a plant with roots deeply valued by Native Americans, has traditionally been a go-to for women's health issues, such as menstrual cramps and menopausal symptoms. The Penobscot people also relied on it for kidney health.

This herb, known for its ability to ease rheumatic aches and pains, including those from rheumatoid arthritis, is also recognized for its potential to calm nerve-related issues like tinnitus. Characterized by its bitter taste and strong smell, black cohosh is a native species to Canada and the eastern United States, thriving in the cooler, shaded areas of woodlands and hedgerows. Nowadays, it's cultivated in Europe and can even be spotted growing wild, having spread from planted specimens. Typically, the seeds are sown, and the roots are collected in the fall.

Uses:

1. Traditionally dubbed "squaw root," black cohosh remains a popular natural solution for menstrual discomfort and low estrogen challenges, along with hot flashes during menopause.

2. For those grappling with inflammatory arthritis linked to menopause, black cohosh offers relief, and it's also employed in managing other rheumatic conditions, such as rheumatoid arthritis.

3. The calming properties of black cohosh make it a versatile remedy, helping manage conditions that range from high blood pressure and whooping cough to tinnitus and asthma.

Preparation:

1. **Black Cohosh Extract:**

- Alcohol Extraction: Black cohosh roots and rhizomes can be dried and soaked in alcohol to create a tincture or liquid extract. This method concentrates the active compounds and can be used medicinally.
- Dosage: Follow the instructions on the tincture bottle or as directed by a healthcare provider.

2. **Black Cohosh Tea:**

- Simple Preparation: Add dried black cohosh roots or rhizomes to boiling water and let steep for 5-10 minutes. Strain and drink.
- Usage: Black cohosh tea is less common due to its bitter taste but can still be consumed for its potential health benefits. If preferred, honey or sugar can be added to sweeten it.

3. **Black Cohosh Capsules or Tablets:**

- Commercial Preparation: Black cohosh supplements are available in capsule or tablet form, often standardized to contain specific concentrations of active compounds.

102 | THE LOST BOOK OF MEDICAL REMEDIES

Follow the dosage instructions on the product label or as directed by a healthcare provider.

Safety and Considerations:

Pregnancy and Breastfeeding: Black cohosh should be avoided during pregnancy and breastfeeding due to its potential effects on hormone levels and uterine contractions.

Liver Health: There have been reports of liver toxicity associated with the use of black cohosh supplements, although these cases are rare. Individuals with liver disease or liver problems should use black cohosh with caution and under the guidance of a healthcare provider.

Allergic Reactions: Some individuals may experience allergic reactions to black cohosh, particularly if they are allergic to other members of the Ranunculaceae family, such as buttercup or pasqueflower.

Echinacea (Purple Coneflower), Echinacea angustifolia

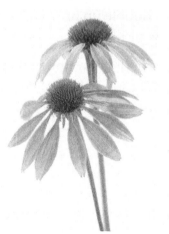

Composition:

• **Primary Components:** Echinacea contains various bioactive compounds, including alkamides, caffeic acid derivatives (such as echinacoside), polysaccharides, and flavonoids.
• **Nutritional Content:** While not typically consumed for its nutritional content, Echinacea does contain small amounts of vitamins and minerals.

Purple Coneflower, also known as Echinacea, is a striking purple bloom resembling a sunflower and is renowned for its medicinal properties. This plant, indigenous to North America, is part of the Asteraceae or Daisy family. It's a popular choice for gardens due to its widespread availability and ease of cultivation. Echinacea naturally thrives in the open, rocky areas of prairies and plains. As a perennial herb, it can reach heights between 6 and 24 inches, with a woody root that often branches out. The plant features one or more rough, hairy stems that are typically straight and unbranched.

The leaves of the Echinacea plant are arranged alternately, simple in structure, and shaped like narrow lances. These leaves, which are toothless and display three clear veins, are spaced out along the lower half of the stem and have a rough, hairy texture. The stems themselves may have a purple or green hue. The flowers of Echinacea are reminiscent of lavender sunflowers, with flowerheads measuring 1 ½ to 3 inches across, sitting atop long stalks that bloom in the summer. The disk flowers within the head are brownish-purple, have five lobes, and are surrounded by stiff bracts that bear yellow pollen. The fruits are tiny, dark, and have four sides, known as achenes.

Uses

1. Echinacea's ability to fight microbes and reduce inflammation makes it a go-to for urinary tract infections (UTIs). It's commonly used alongside goldenseal root, but it's important to avoid both if you have an autoimmune condition.

2. This plant is a powerhouse with antibiotic, antifungal, antiviral properties, and it's known to give the immune system a boost. It's effective against various infections and can be used both on the skin and taken internally.

3. If you've been bitten by a spider or stung by an insect, Echinacea can help. It's great at neutralizing toxins and easing pain. There are also claims that it can be beneficial for snakebites due to its strong anti-inflammatory effects.

4. When it comes to the common cold and flu, Echinacea can lessen the blow. Starting Echinacea extract or tea right when you feel under the weather can speed up recovery significantly. Some say you can get better up to 4 days sooner compared to those who don't use it (and the same is true for blue elderberry). For optimal results, double up on your first day's dose three times and continue with regular doses throughout your illness.

5. Echinacea is also a friend to those with allergies, as it helps modulate the immune system. It's particularly useful for easing asthma attacks. While it's not a cure for asthma, it can reduce the intensity of an attack and aid in recovery. It's also handy for treating bronchitis.

Preparation:

1. Echinacea Tea:

- Simple Preparation: Add dried Echinacea roots, leaves, or flowers to boiling water and let steep for 5-10 minutes. Strain and drink.
- Usage: Echinacea tea is commonly consumed to support immune function and overall well-being, particularly during cold and flu season. It has a slightly bitter taste and can be sweetened with honey or sugar if desired.

2. Echinacea Tincture:

- Alcohol Extraction: Echinacea roots, leaves, or flowers can be soaked in alcohol to create a tincture. This method concentrates the active compounds and can be used medicinally.

- Dosage: Follow the instructions on the tincture bottle or as directed by a healthcare provider.

3. Echinacea Capsules or Tablets:

- Commercial Preparation: Echinacea supplements are available in capsule or tablet form, often standardized to contain specific concentrations of active compounds. Follow the dosage instructions on the product label or as directed by a healthcare provider.

Safety and Considerations:

Allergic Reactions: Some individuals may be allergic to Echinacea, particularly those who are allergic to plants in the Asteraceae family, such as ragweed, daisies, and marigolds.

Pregnancy and Breastfeeding: While Echinacea is generally considered safe for most individuals, pregnant and breastfeeding women should consult with a healthcare provider before using it as a herbal remedy.

Autoimmune Disorders: Echinacea should be used cautiously by people with autoimmune illnesses since it may boost the immune system and worsen symptoms.

Cinchona, Cinchona spp.

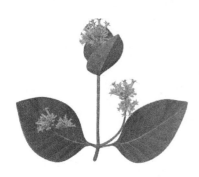

Composition:

- Primary Components: Cinchona bark contains various alkaloids, with quinine being the most well-known and studied. Other alkaloids found in cinchona bark include quinidine, cinchonidine, and cinchonine.
- Nutritional Content: While not typically consumed for its nutritional content, cinchona bark contains various bioactive compounds with medicinal properties.

Cinchona is renowned for being the plant that gives us quinine, historically the most popular treatment for malaria around the globe. A Jesuit missionary first recorded its use in Peru back in 1633. Beyond its antimalarial properties, cinchona is also tapped for its benefits in treating fevers and aiding digestion. Medicinal uses extend to several species like C. calisaya, C. ledgeriana, and C. officinalis. Originally from the mountainous tropics of South America, particularly Peru, cinchona cultivation has spread to India, Java, and certain African regions. These trees are typically grown from cuttings planted in the late spring. Harvesting involves removing and sun-drying the bark from trees that are between six and eight years old. Each year, around 8,000 tons of cinchona bark are produced globally.

Uses

1. In Peru, locals have been using cinchona for ages to combat fevers, digestive issues, and infections. It remains a go-to natural remedy for these ailments today.

2. Around 1790, Samuel Hahnemann, the guy who came up with homeopathy, made his first homeopathic concoction using cinchona.

3. Before the First World War, quinine, derived from cinchona, was the go-to fix for malaria. With malaria parasites becoming resistant to chloroquine in the 1960s, quinine made a comeback in malaria prevention and treatment. It's also handy for other feverish conditions.

4. Need a digestive pick-me-up? Cinchona's bitter qualities are great for getting those digestive juices flowing and kick-starting your appetite.

5. Got a sore throat? Cinchona works wonders as a gargle to soothe and fight infection.

6. The herb isn't just for throats; it's a natural remedy for cramps, including those pesky night cramps, and it even eases arthritis pain.

7. Over in India, cinchona is the go-to herb for a variety of health issues, from sciatica and dysentery to balancing kapha-related problems.

Preparation:

1. Cinchona Bark Tea:
   - Simple Preparation: Add dried cinchona bark to boiling water and let steep for 10-15 minutes. Strain and drink.
   - Usage: Cinchona bark tea is traditionally used to treat malaria and is believed to have antipyretic (fever-reducing) and analgesic (pain-relieving) properties. It has a bitter taste and may be sweetened with honey or sugar if desired.

2. Cinchona Tincture:
   - Alcohol Extraction: Cinchona bark can be soaked in alcohol to create a tincture. This method concentrates the active compounds and can be used medicinally.
   - Dosage: Follow the instructions on the tincture bottle or as directed by a healthcare provider.

3. Cinchona Capsules or Tablets:
   - Commercial Preparation: Cinchona supplements are available in capsule or tablet form, often standardized to contain specific concentrations of quinine or other alkaloids. Follow the dosage instructions on the product label or as directed by a healthcare provider.

Safety and Considerations:

Quinine Toxicity: Cinchona bark and quinine supplements should be used with caution due to the potential risk of quinine toxicity, which can cause adverse effects such as cinchonism (nausea, vomiting, tinnitus, dizziness) and, in severe cases, cardiac arrhythmias and death. Dosages should be carefully monitored, and it's important to consult with a healthcare provider before using cinchona bark or quinine supplements.

Pregnancy and Breastfeeding: Cinchona bark and quinine supplements should be avoided during pregnancy and breastfeeding unless specifically prescribed by a healthcare provider, as they may pose risks to the developing fetus or nursing infant.

Drug Interactions: Quinine may interact with certain medications, including anticoagulants, anticonvulsants, and medications metabolized by the liver. Consult with a healthcare provider before using cinchona bark or quinine supplements if you are taking medication.

Elecampane, Inula helenium

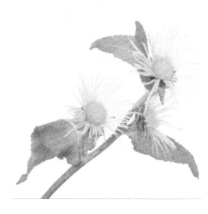

Composition:

- Primary Components: Elecampane contains various bioactive compounds, including sesquiterpene lactones (such as alantolactone and isoalantolactone), inulin (a type of soluble fiber), and essential oils.
- Nutritional Content: While not typically consumed for its nutritional content, elecampane root contains small amounts of vitamins and minerals.

Elecampane, part of the sunflower tribe, goes by various names like horse-heal, wild sunflower, and elfdock. There's a myth that it grew from where Helen of Troy's tears landed. The Celts revered it, linking it to the mystical fairy realm. You'll find it thriving in damp, shadowy spots, and it's widely grown and has taken root in the eastern US, dotting pastures and roadsides, especially on slopes facing east and south. It stands tall, reaching up to 6 feet, with large, rough leaves that come in shapes like egg, elliptical, or lance. The lower leaves have stems, but the upper ones don't. Each leaf can be a foot or more long and about 5 inches across, with a fuzzy green top and a soft white underside. The flower heads are sizable, up to 3 inches across, with a sunny yellow color and look like a fuller version of a sunflower. Elecampane flowers from June through August, and its roots are brown, aromatic, and branch out underground. They're thick, sticky, and have a bitter taste with a hint of camphor and a floral scent.

Uses

1. Got a cough or dealing with asthma, bronchitis, whooping cough, or tuberculosis? Elecampane root can help! It's an expectorant, meaning it helps break up mucus, making your cough more effective. It's not for dry coughs, though. It calms the lining of your bronchial tubes, eases swelling and irritation, cleans out your lungs, and battles bugs in your respiratory system. If your cough is really bugging you, take small doses often. It's also a buddy for your lungs if you've got asthma, much like mullein.

2. If you're watching your blood sugar or managing type 2 diabetes, elecampane's high inulin content is your friend. Inulin takes it slow with sugar metabolism, keeping those blood sugar spikes in check and helping with insulin resistance. Plus, it might even tone down inflammation that comes with diabetes.

3. This plant is also a champ at kicking out unwanted guests like intestinal parasites. Say goodbye to hookworms, roundworms, threadworms, and whipworms.

4. There are compounds in elecampane, called alantolactone and isoalantolactone, that show promise in triggering cell death in certain cancer cells.

5. Beyond its respiratory benefits, elecampane is a star for digestive issues. It warms, drains, and adds a bitter kick. Use it for when your digestion feels off, you're not soaking up nutrients well, your appetite's down, you've got too much mucus or gas, or your digestion just feels tired. It boosts digestion and nutrient absorption, which is great if you're not getting enough nourishment. Plus, it can help with nausea and diarrhea.

Preparation:

1. Elecampane Tea:

- Simple Preparation: Add dried elecampane roots to boiling water and let steep for 10-15 minutes. Strain and drink.
- Usage: Elecampane tea is traditionally used to support respiratory health and relieve symptoms of coughs, bronchitis, and congestion. It has a slightly bitter and aromatic taste.

2. Elecampane Tincture:

- Alcohol Extraction: Elecampane roots can be soaked in alcohol to create a tincture. This method concentrates the active compounds and can be used medicinally.
- Dosage: Follow the instructions on the tincture bottle or as directed by a healthcare provider.

3. Elecampane Syrup:

- Sweetened Preparation: Elecampane root decoction can be mixed with honey or sugar to create a soothing syrup for coughs and respiratory congestion.
- Usage: Elecampane syrup is often used as a natural remedy for coughs, sore throats, and respiratory infections. It can be taken by the spoonful as needed.

Safety and Considerations:

Allergic Reactions: Some individuals may be allergic to elecampane or other plants in the Asteraceae family, such as ragweed, daisies, and marigolds. Use caution if you have known allergies to these plants.

Pregnancy and Breastfeeding: Elecampane is generally considered safe when consumed in moderate amounts as food, but pregnant and breastfeeding women should consult with a healthcare provider before using it as a medicinal herb or supplement.

Drug Interactions: Elecampane may interact with certain medications, particularly anticoagulants and medications metabolized by the liver. Consult with a healthcare provider before using elecampane supplements if you are taking medication.

Cinnamon, Cinnamomum spp.

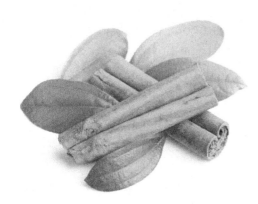

Composition:

- Primary Components: Cinnamon contains various bioactive compounds, including cinnamaldehyde, cinnamic acid, and cinnamyl alcohol. These compounds give cinnamon its distinct flavor and aroma.
- Nutritional Content: Cinnamon is a good source of antioxidants, such as polyphenols, and contains small amounts of vitamins and minerals, including manganese, calcium, and iron.

Cinnamon holds a prestigious spot as one of the most significant spices in the world, with its roots tracing back to ancient medicinal practices, first documented in the sacred Jewish text, the Torah. This spice boasts a storied past, particularly in India and Southeast Asia, before making its way to Egypt around 2000 BCE and eventually to Europe by 500 BCE. Traditionally, people turned to cinnamon to combat colds, flu, and digestive issues, but today, it's also popular for its ability to help regulate blood sugar levels. Originating from India and Sri Lanka, true cinnamon (C. zeylanicum) thrives in tropical forests up to an altitude of 1,600 feet (500 meters). Cultivation now extends to the Philippines and the

Caribbean. The trees are grown from cuttings and are pruned to the ground every other year. The following year, the bark is harvested from the new shoots, and the inner layer is dried in the sun, curling into the familiar quills we know.

Uses:

1. Cinnamon has long been cherished as a warming herb, especially for treating "cold" conditions and is often paired with ginger (Zingiber officinale) to boost circulation and warm the body. It's a go-to remedy for flu-like symptoms and serves as an effective mouthwash for oral thrush.

2. During recovery from illness, cinnamon is a mild yet supportive herb that aids both digestion and blood flow. It's particularly helpful for those feeling weak or in the process of recuperating.

3. For menstrual relief, cinnamon can ease cramps and help regulate menstrual flow, lessening heavy periods and encouraging flow when scant. It's also beneficial for managing PCOS (polycystic ovary syndrome) by lowering insulin and balancing estrogen levels.

4. Cinnamon plays a key role in maintaining healthy blood sugar levels and preventing insulin resistance, a precursor to diabetes. A common recommendation for those managing diabetes or metabolic syndrome is to consume 3 teaspoons of cinnamon powder daily for four months, as part of a comprehensive health plan.

5. Cinnamon has always been a go-to for soothing digestive ailments, providing relief from nausea, indigestion, gas, as well as colic and diarrhea. Its antifungal properties also make it useful in addressing imbalances in gut bacteria.

Preparation:

1. Cinnamon Powder:

- Simple Preparation: Cinnamon sticks or quills can be ground into a fine powder using a spice grinder or mortar and pestle.
- Usage: Cinnamon powder is commonly used as a spice in cooking and baking. It adds warmth and sweetness to dishes and can be used in both sweet and savory recipes.

2. Cinnamon Sticks:

- Whole Preparation: Cinnamon sticks or quills can be used whole to infuse flavor into hot beverages, such as tea, coffee, or mulled cider.
- Usage: Cinnamon sticks are also used as a decorative garnish in dishes and beverages. They can be added to soups, stews, and curries during cooking to impart flavor.

3. Cinnamon Oil:

- Extraction Process: Cinnamon oil can be extracted from cinnamon bark using steam distillation or solvent extraction methods.
- Usage: Cinnamon oil is used in aromatherapy for its warming and stimulating properties. It can also be used as a flavoring agent in foods, beverages, and oral care products.

Safety and Considerations:

Cassia vs. Ceylon Cinnamon: There are two main types of cinnamon available: cassia cinnamon (Cinnamomum cassia) and Ceylon cinnamon (Cinnamomum verum). Cassia cinnamon contains higher levels of coumarin, which may be harmful in large doses. Ceylon cinnamon is considered safer for regular consumption.

Allergic Reactions: Some individuals may be allergic to cinnamon or experience irritation when applied topically. Use caution if you have known allergies to cinnamon or other spices.

Pregnancy and Breastfeeding: Cinnamon is generally considered safe when consumed in moderate amounts as food, but pregnant and breastfeeding women should avoid excessive consumption of cinnamon supplements or extracts.

Evening Primrose, Oenothera biennis

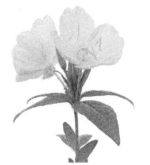

Composition:

- **Primary Components:** Evening primrose seeds are rich in gamma-linolenic acid (GLA), an omega-6 fatty acid, as well as linoleic acid and other essential fatty acids.
- **Nutritional Content:** Evening primrose seeds also contain vitamins, minerals, and antioxidants, including vitamin E.

Evening primrose, also known as evening star or sun drop, is a plant that blooms as the day fades, its blossoms unfurling in the twilight. This plant, native to eastern and central North America and now found throughout Europe, belongs to the Onagraceae family. The species Oenothera biennis is a two-year grower, with the first year's leaves reaching up to 10 inches long, shaped like a lance, edged with teeth, and grouped into a rosette. Come the second year, it shoots up a stem with leaves spiraling up its rough, sometimes purple-tinged surface, growing 3 to 6 feet tall. From June through October, it bears bright yellow flowers that shy away from the day's heat, each with four petals, spanning 1 to 2 inches across, and clustering at the stem's end. These sweet-smelling blooms are short-lived, lasting just a day or two, followed by slender seedpods.

Uses

1. It's a whiz at smoothing out hormonal ups and downs in women, tackling PMS discomforts like sore breasts, bloating, and mood swings, not to mention helping with PCOS, fertility, and regulating menstrual cycles. It's also a buddy during menopause, easing hot flashes and restless nights.

2. Evening primrose steps up to the plate against hormonal hair loss in both men and women, encouraging hair to stick around and sometimes even make a comeback. For the best shot at results, mix it up both inside and out, pairing it with a little rosemary oil scalp massage.

3. If you're dealing with rheumatoid arthritis or osteoporosis, evening primrose oil can be your go-to. It's like a balm for inflammation, easing aches and helping bones hold onto their strength by balancing bone-weakening hormones. Plus, it plays nice with calcium and fish oil for an extra boost.

4. Got a tummy in turmoil? The plant's bark and leaves come to the rescue with their soothing, astringent powers, putting the brakes on those pesky muscle spasms and setting the stage for happier digestion.

5. For those with a cough that just won't quit, evening primrose steps in as an expectorant. A homemade flower syrup can make whooping cough a little easier to handle, especially for the kiddos.

6. Keeping evening primrose oil in your routine can be a heart-helper, nudging down cholesterol and blood pressure. But remember, it's a slow and steady kind of deal, not a quick fix.

7. And for folks with diabetes feeling the sting of nerve pain, evening primrose oil might just be the relief you're looking for.

Preparation:

1. Evening Primrose Oil:

- Cold-Press Extraction: Evening primrose seeds are cold-pressed to extract the oil, preserving its nutritional integrity.
- Usage: Evening primrose oil is available as a dietary supplement in capsule or liquid form. It can also be used topically as a skin moisturizer or in homemade skincare products.

2. Evening Primrose Tea:

- Simple Preparation: Evening primrose leaves and flowers can be steeped in hot water to make tea.

- Usage: Evening primrose tea is less common but may still be consumed for its potential health benefits, such as promoting relaxation and relieving menstrual cramps.

Safety and Considerations:

Allergic Reactions: Some individuals may be allergic to evening primrose or other plants in the Onagraceae family. Use caution if you have known allergies to these plants.

Pregnancy and Breastfeeding: Evening primrose oil is generally considered safe for most adults when used in moderate amounts, but pregnant and breastfeeding women should consult with a healthcare provider before using it as a supplement.

Blood Thinning: Evening primrose oil may have mild blood-thinning effects due to its omega-6 fatty acids. Use caution if you are taking blood-thinning medications or have a bleeding disorder.

Lemon, Citrus limon

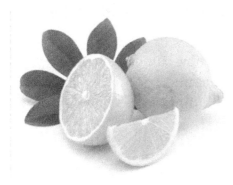

Composition:

•**Primary Components:** Lemons are rich in vitamin C, citric acid, flavonoids, and other antioxidants. They also contain small amounts of vitamins, minerals, and dietary fiber.

•**Nutritional Content:** Lemons are low in calories but high in vitamin C, providing about 64% of the recommended daily intake per 100 grams.

Lemon is one of the most important and versatile natural medicines for home use. It's a common snack that doubles as a medicine because of its high vitamin C content, which boosts immunity against infection and is beneficial for colds and the flu. It is taken as a preventative for many conditions, including stomach infections, circulatory problems, and arteriosclerosis (thickening of the arterial walls). Thought to be native to India, lemon trees were first grown in Europe in the 2nd century cE and are now cultivated in Mediterranean and subtropical climates worldwide. Propagated from seed in spring, they prefer well-drained soil and plenty of sun. The fruit is harvested in winter when the vitamin C content is at its highest.

Uses

1. Spanish popular medicine ascribes so many medicinal uses to lemon that whole books have been written about it.

2. Despite its acid content, once digested, lemon has an alkaline effect within the body, making it useful in rheumatic conditions where acidity is a contributory factor. The volatile oil is antiseptic and antibacterial. In addition to being antioxidants, bioflavonoids also help prevent varicose veins and easy bruising by strengthening the inner lining of blood vessels, particularly veins and capillaries.

3. Preventative Lemon is a valuable preventative medicine. Its antiseptic and cleansing actions make it useful for those prone to arteriosclerosis, and to infections and fevers (especially of the stomach, liver, and intestines). Its ability to strengthen blood vessel walls helps prevent circulatory disorders and bleeding gums. Lemon is also useful as a general tonic for many chronic illnesses. It is a food that promotes overall health above everything else.

4. Lemon juice is good for colds, flu, and chest infections. It stimulates liver detoxification, improves the appetite, and helps ease stomach acidity, ulcers, arthritis, gout, and rheumatism. As a gargle, lemon juice is helpful for sore throats, gingivitis, and mouth ulcers. Externally, lemon juice can be applied directly to acne, athlete's foot, chilblains, insect stings, ringworm, sunburn, and warts.

5. The whole fruit, especially the pith, treats arteriosclerosis, weak capillaries, and varicose veins.

Lemon (Citrus limon) is a citrus fruit native to South Asia but now cultivated in many parts of the world for its culinary and medicinal uses. Rich in vitamin C and other nutrients, lemons are prized for their refreshing flavor and versatile applications. Here's how to prepare and use lemons:

Preparation:

1. Lemon Juice:

- Simple Extraction: Squeeze fresh lemon juice from ripe lemons using a citrus juicer or by hand.
- Usage: Lemon juice is commonly used as a flavoring agent in cooking, baking, and beverages. It adds a tangy, citrusy flavor to dishes and can be used to enhance the taste of salads, marinades, sauces, and cocktails.

2. Lemon Zest:

- Grated Peel: Use a fine grater or zester to remove the outer zest of lemons, avoiding the bitter white pith.

- Usage: Lemon zest adds a bright, aromatic flavor to dishes and can be used in both sweet and savory recipes. It is often added to baked goods, dressings, marinades, and desserts.

3. Preserved Lemons:

- Salt-Preserved: Lemons can be preserved in salt to create a tangy, flavorful condiment used in Middle Eastern and North African cuisine.
- Usage: Preserved lemons add a unique depth of flavor to dishes such as tagines, salads, and couscous. They can also be used to make sauces and dressings.

Safety and Considerations:

Citrus Allergies: Some individuals may be allergic to citrus fruits, including lemons. If you have known allergies to citrus fruits, use caution when consuming lemons or products containing lemon ingredients.

Dental Health: Citric acid in lemon juice can erode tooth enamel over time, leading to tooth sensitivity and decay. Rinse your mouth with water after consuming lemon juice and avoid brushing your teeth immediately to minimize enamel damage.

Skin Sensitivity: Direct contact with lemon juice on the skin can cause photosensitivity and irritation, particularly when exposed to sunlight. Avoid applying lemon juice to sensitive or sun-exposed areas of the skin.

Fennel, Foeniculum vulgare

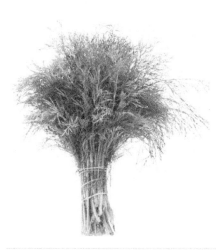

Composition:

- **Primary Components:** Fennel contains various phytochemicals, including anethole (responsible for its licorice-like flavor), flavonoids, phenolic compounds, and volatile oils.
- **Nutritional Content:** Fennel is low in calories but rich in fiber, vitamins (such as vitamin C, vitamin K, and folate), and minerals (such as potassium and manganese).

Fennel is a popular veggie in the same family as celery, carrots, and parsley, known as Apiaceae or Umbelliferae. It's got this cool licorice taste and smells amazing. You can spot it all over the US and Canada. I've got it growing in my backyard, but it's also pretty common by the roads, along rivers, and in fields. It's a perennial herb that blooms and sports these cute yellow flowers. It kinda resembles dill, but with a bulb at the base. Its leaves are super delicate, even more so than dill, and the plant stands tall and green, reaching up to eight feet. The leaves are really thin, and the bulb is formed by leafy branches spreading out from the stem. It flowers in clusters, each with loads of tiny yellow blooms. The seeds are little guys, grooved and about a fifth to a third of an inch long.

Uses

1. Sip on some seed-infused tea after meals to sort out any tummy troubles like indigestion, heartburn, or gas. It's a champ for constipation and stomach aches too. Plus, tossing some seeds into your cooking can help with digestion.

2. Moms dealing with a colicky baby can drink this tea to soothe the little one and boost milk production. Babies who aren't nursing can have a bit of the tea to calm colic symptoms.

3. For regulating periods and hormonal issues, Fennel Seed Tea is your go-to. It can ease cramps, PMS, and other menstrual discomforts, thanks to its estrogen-like compounds.

4. Got a sore throat or achy gums? Gargling with this tea can kick the pain and fight off the infection.

5. If you're battling urinary issues like infections or kidney stones, try a boiled concoction made from fennel root.

6. As a potent diuretic and cleanser, fennel can help your body get rid of toxins and extra fluids. Drinking the tea up to three times a day can help detoxify your system.

7. To boost your eyesight, include fennel in your meals. And for eye problems like inflammation or infections, using the tea as an eyewash can be really beneficial. It's great for treating conditions like conjunctivitis too.

Preparation:

1. Fennel Bulb:

- **Trimming:** Remove the stalks and fronds from the fennel bulb. Trim the base and any tough or discolored outer layers.
- Slicing: Slice the bulb vertically into thin slices or chop it into smaller pieces, depending on the recipe.

- Usage: Fennel bulbs can be eaten raw in salads, slaws, and crudité platters, or cooked by roasting, grilling, sautéing, or braising. They have a crisp texture and sweet, anise-like flavor when raw, which becomes milder and sweeter when cooked.

2. Fennel Seeds:

- Harvesting: Fennel seeds are harvested from the dried fruits (schizocarps) of the fennel plant.
- Storage: Store whole fennel seeds in an airtight container in a cool, dry place away from direct sunlight to maintain their flavor and aroma.
- Usage: Fennel seeds are used as a spice in cooking and baking, particularly in Indian, Middle Eastern, and Mediterranean cuisines. They can be toasted, ground, or infused into dishes to add a warm, aromatic flavor reminiscent of licorice.

3. Fennel Fronds:

- Trimming: Separate the feathery fronds from the stalks and discard any tough or woody parts.
- Usage: Fennel fronds can be used as a garnish in salads, soups, and seafood dishes, adding a delicate, herbal flavor and visual appeal. They can also be incorporated into sauces, dressings, and pestos for added freshness and aroma.

Safety and Considerations:

Allergic Reactions: Some individuals may be allergic to fennel or other plants in the Apiaceae family, such as carrots, celery, and parsley. Use caution if you have known allergies to these plants.

Pregnancy and Breastfeeding: Fennel is generally considered safe for most adults when consumed in moderate amounts as food, but pregnant and breastfeeding women should consult with a healthcare provider before using fennel supplements or extracts due to limited safety data.

Medication Interactions: Fennel may interact with certain medications, including blood thinners, estrogen-based medications, and medications metabolized by the liver. Consult with a healthcare provider before using fennel supplements or extracts if you are taking medication.

Codonopsis, Codonopsis pilosula

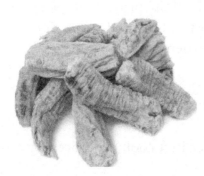

Composition:

• **Primary Components:** Codonopsis contains various bioactive compounds, including polysaccharides, alkaloids, saponins, flavonoids, and polyacetylenes.

• **Nutritional Content:** Codonopsis root is rich in carbohydrates, dietary fiber, and minerals, such as calcium, magnesium, and potassium.

Codonopsis holds a revered spot in the realm of traditional Chinese medicine, serving as a soothing strengthener that boosts energy, enhances overall physical and mental health, and assists the body in managing stress. It's akin to ginseng in its adaptogenic effects, though it's gentler and doesn't last as long. For those who find ginseng too potent, codonopsis is the go-to alternative, and it's often swapped for ginseng in herbal mixtures. This plant is indigenous to China's northeast, flourishing especially in the Shanxi and Szechuan areas. You can grow it from seeds in either spring or fall, and the roots are ready for harvest in the fall, after the top parts have withered away.

Uses

1. It's all about invigorating the body's qi, or life force, as well as bolstering the lungs and spleen in Chinese medicine. It boosts overall vigor and helps keep the body's metabolism in check. As a mild tonic, it rejuvenates the entire system.

2. Codonopsis is the herb of choice for those feeling weak, worn out, or struggling with digestive troubles like lack of appetite, nausea, and diarrhea. It's known to nurture the stomach's yin without causing excess dampness and to fortify the spleen without drying it out. It's especially helpful for long-term conditions linked to a deficiency in spleen qi.

3. Interestingly, codonopsis is recommended for folks dealing with stress and "false fire" issues such as stiff necks, headaches, irritability, and high blood pressure. Stronger adaptogens like ginseng might worsen these symptoms, but codonopsis is particularly good at calming adrenaline spikes and the stress that comes with them.

4. In China, nursing moms take it regularly to boost milk production and as a nourishing tonic to "build strong blood."

5. It's also great for clearing out excess mucus from the lungs, making it handy for respiratory issues like breathlessness and asthma.

Preparation:

1. Codonopsis Decoction:

- Simple Preparation: Simmer dried Codonopsis root slices in water to make a decoction.
- Usage: Codonopsis decoction is traditionally used in traditional Chinese medicine (TCM) to tonify Qi (vital energy), nourish the spleen and stomach, and promote overall vitality and well-being. It is often consumed as a tea or added to soups, stews, and herbal formulations.

2. Codonopsis Tincture:

- Alcohol Extraction: Codonopsis root can be soaked in alcohol to create a tincture.
- Usage: Codonopsis tincture is a concentrated form of the herb that can be taken orally by adding a few drops to water or juice. It is believed to have similar therapeutic effects as the decoction but in a more convenient and portable form.

Safety and Considerations:

Allergic Reactions: Some individuals may be allergic to Codonopsis or other plants in the Campanulaceae family. Use caution if you have known allergies to these plants.

Pregnancy and Breastfeeding: Codonopsis is generally considered safe for most adults when consumed in moderate amounts as food or medicine, but pregnant and breastfeeding women should consult with a healthcare provider before using Codonopsis supplements or extracts due to limited safety data.

Medication Interactions: Codonopsis may interact with certain medications, including blood thinners, immunosuppressants, and medications metabolized by the liver. Consult with a healthcare provider before using Codonopsis supplements or extracts if you are taking medication.

Feverfew, Tanacetum parthenium

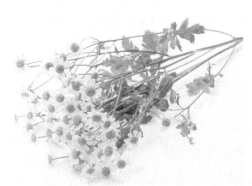

Composition:

- Primary Components: Feverfew contains various bioactive compounds, including sesquiterpene lactones (such as parthenolide), flavonoids, volatile oils, and other phytochemicals.
- Nutritional Content: Feverfew is not typically consumed for its nutritional content but may contain small amounts of vitamins and minerals.

Feverfew, a popular herb for combating migraines, thrives in rocky, disturbed soils and along roadsides. It's also grown in various home gardens, both for herbs and decoration. Known by several names like Chrysanthemum parthenium, wild chamomile, or bachelor's buttons, it belongs to the Aster/Daisy family. This bushy plant stands about 1 to 3 feet tall and features leafy round stems sprouting from a taproot. Its yellow-green leaves are intricately divided, with the upper ones more lobed and toothed. They emit a distinctively bitter scent and flavor. Come summer, feverfew blooms with tiny daisy-like flowers, sporting a flat yellow center surrounded by short white petals, distinguishing it from the conical centers of chamomiles.

Uses:

1. Regular intake of feverfew can help prevent migraine attacks, similar to butterbur, but consistency is key. Its potential benefits include anti-inflammatory properties, easing muscle contractions, pain relief, and reducing blood platelet clumping. Plus, ongoing research might reveal even more ways it helps.

2. The herb's name stems from its historical use in fever treatment. A hot cup of Feverfew Tea can help reduce fever and soothe the discomforts of colds and flu due to its anti-inflammatory and pain-relieving effects. For baby colic or discomfort in toddlers, a few drops of a cool infusion might do the trick.

3. Feverfew also acts as a uterine stimulant and painkiller, especially effective for easing painful menstrual cramps and inducing menstruation.

Preparation:

1. Feverfew Tea:

- Simple Preparation: Steep dried Feverfew leaves or flowers in hot water to make a tea.
- Usage: Feverfew tea is traditionally used to alleviate symptoms of headaches, migraines, fever, and inflammation. It has a bitter taste, so it may be sweetened with honey or other natural sweeteners if desired.

2. Feverfew Tincture:

- Alcohol Extraction: Feverfew leaves and flowers can be soaked in alcohol to create a tincture.
- Usage: Feverfew tincture is a concentrated form of the herb that can be taken orally by adding a few drops to water or juice. It is believed to have similar therapeutic effects as the tea but in a more concentrated form.

Safety and Considerations:

Allergic Reactions: Some individuals may be allergic to Feverfew or other plants in the Asteraceae family, such as ragweed, daisies, and marigolds. Use caution if you have known allergies to these plants.

Pregnancy and Breastfeeding: Feverfew is not recommended for use during pregnancy or breastfeeding due to its potential to stimulate uterine contractions and cause miscarriage. It may also pass into breast milk and affect nursing infants.

Medication Interactions: Feverfew may interact with certain medications, including blood thinners, nonsteroidal anti-inflammatory drugs (NSAIDs), and medications metabolized by the liver. Consult with a healthcare provider before using Feverfew supplements or extracts if you are taking medication.

Coleus, Plectranthus barbatus

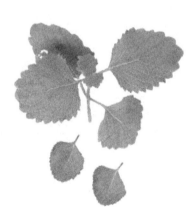

Composition:

- Primary Components: Coleus contains forskolin, a bioactive compound found in the roots of the plant. Forskolin is believed to have various pharmacological effects, including vasodilation, bronchodilation, and anti-inflammatory properties.
- Nutritional Content: Coleus is not typically consumed for its nutritional content but may contain small amounts of vitamins, minerals, and antioxidants.

Originating from India, coleus is a plant traditionally utilized in local folk remedies rather than in the established Ayurvedic system. It's commonly used as a natural solution for digestive issues. The plant gained recognition in the West when forskolin, one of its components, was extracted in the 1970s. Subsequent research by a collaboration between Indian and German scientists revealed forskolin's effectiveness in treating a variety of ailments, such as heart failure, glaucoma, and bronchial asthma. The coleus plant thrives on

India's arid slopes and the lower regions of the Himalayas, as well as in other warm locations like Nepal, Sri Lanka, Myanmar, and parts of eastern Africa. Once a favored decorative plant in the 19th century, coleus is now extensively cultivated in Gujarat, India, mainly for its inclusion in pickles, with an annual harvest of roughly 980 tons. Propagation is through stem cuttings or splitting the roots in the warmer seasons, and the plant does best in well-drained soil with some sun or light shade. Harvesting of the roots and leaves takes place in the fall.

Uses:

1. It's a go-to herb for a variety of digestive troubles in India, offering relief from gas, bloating, and stomach discomfort.

2. As a cardiac and circulatory booster, coleus is applied to manage congestive heart failure and enhance blood flow to the heart and brain.

3. Thanks to its antispasmodic properties, coleus is beneficial for respiratory issues, including asthma and bronchitis.

4. Applied externally, coleus helps in managing glaucoma by relieving the excessive pressure that can impair vision if left untreated.

5. Coleus has also entered the market as a potential weight-loss supplement. The claim is that it boosts cellular metabolism, which could aid in shedding pounds. However, there's no concrete evidence to back this claim, although it might assist if weight gain is linked to suboptimal thyroid function.

Preparation:

1. Coleus Extract:

- Extraction Process: Forskolin is extracted from the roots of Coleus plants using solvent extraction or other methods.
- Usage: Coleus extract is available in various forms, including capsules, tablets, and liquid extracts. Its possible health benefits have led to its widespread use as a dietary supplement.

Safety and Considerations:

Allergic Reactions: Some individuals may be allergic to Coleus or other plants in the Lamiaceae family, such as mint, basil, and oregano. Use caution if you have known allergies to these plants.

Pregnancy and Breastfeeding: Coleus extract is not recommended for use during pregnancy or breastfeeding due to limited safety data. Forskolin may stimulate uterine contractions and cause miscarriage in pregnant women.

Medication Interactions: Coleus extract may interact with certain medications, including blood thinners, antihypertensive drugs, and medications metabolized by the liver. Consult with a healthcare provider before using Coleus supplements or extracts if you are taking medication.

Myrrh, Commiphora myrrha

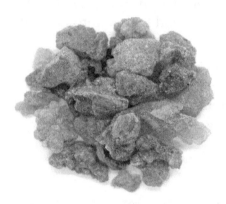

Composition:

- **Primary Components:** Myrrh contains various bioactive compounds, including resin, essential oils, and gums. The main active constituents of myrrh include sesquiterpenes, triterpenoids, and volatile oils.
- **Nutritional Content:** Myrrh is not typically consumed for its nutritional content but may contain trace amounts of minerals and other nutrients.

Myrrh has been treasured for its role in perfumery, incense creation, and the preservation of the deceased. Symbolizing affliction, it was famously presented to baby Jesus by the Magi. Recognized as one of the earliest medicinal substances, myrrh was a staple in the medical practices of the Egyptians. It's particularly good for treating oral and throat issues due to its astringent and somewhat bitter flavor, and it's also beneficial for various skin conditions. This resin-producing plant is indigenous to the arid regions of northeast Africa, with Somalia being a primary source. Nowadays, it can also be found in Ethiopia, Saudi Arabia, India, Iran, and Thailand, thriving in sunny, well-drained environments. Myrrh is grown from seeds in the spring or from cuttings at the end of the growth cycle, and its valuable resin is harvested from slashed branches before being dried for use.

Uses

1. Myrrh is a go-to natural treatment for sore throats, mouth ulcers, and gum disease due to its astringent and potent antiseptic properties. Since it doesn't dissolve in water, it's typically used in tincture or oil form and then diluted. The resulting mouthwash or gargle can quickly alleviate discomfort, despite its strong bitterness. Myrrh is also effective against infections in the digestive system and promotes healing, particularly with conditions like gastric ulcers.

2. In the realm of Ayurvedic healing, myrrh is seen as a rejuvenating and sensual enhancer and is believed to purify the blood. It's credited with boosting mental acuity and is also used to address menstrual irregularities and discomfort.

3. Often overlooked for skin issues, myrrh can be a powerful remedy for acne, boils, and other inflammatory skin conditions. Its drying and mildly numbing effects have even led to its adoption in Germany for treating bedsores associated with prosthetic devices.

Preparation:

1. Myrrh Resin:

- Harvesting: Myrrh resin is obtained by making incisions in the bark of the Commiphora myrrha tree and allowing the sap to ooze out and harden into resinous tears.
- Processing: The hardened resin tears are collected, cleaned, and dried to preserve their aroma and medicinal properties.
- Usage: Myrrh resin can be burned as incense, dissolved in alcohol to make tinctures, infused into oils for topical use, or ground into powders for various applications.

Safety and Considerations:

Allergic Reactions: Some individuals may be allergic to myrrh or other resins. Use caution if you have known allergies to these substances.

Pregnancy and Breastfeeding: Myrrh is not recommended for use during pregnancy or breastfeeding due to limited safety data. It may stimulate uterine contractions and cause miscarriage in pregnant women.

Medication Interactions: Myrrh may interact with certain medications, including blood thinners, anticoagulants, and medications metabolized by the liver. Consult with a healthcare provider before using myrrh supplements or extracts if you are taking medication.

Goldenrod, Solidago spp.

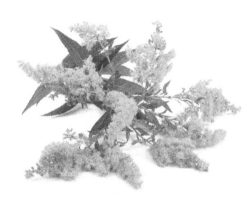

Composition:

- **Primary Components:** Goldenrod contains various bioactive compounds, including flavonoids, saponins, tannins, and essential oils. The specific composition may vary depending on the species and growing conditions.
- **Nutritional Content:** Goldenrod is not typically consumed for its nutritional content but may contain small amounts of vitamins, minerals, and antioxidants.

Goldenrods are a group of around 100 species that thrive across North America in places like meadows and prairies. My go-to is Solidago canadensis, the most widespread type in North America, belonging to the Aster/Daisy Family. It's also called goldruthe and woundwort. Despite getting a bad rap for causing allergies, it's usually not the culprit—ragweed is often to blame. Goldenrods are bee-pollinated and don't scatter pollen in the air like ragweed does. Plus, they can actually help with ragweed allergies. You'll spot them in open spaces and by trails, identifiable by their smell, taste, and look—tall with bunches of yellow flowers. Crush their leaves and you'll get a salty, balsamic scent. While any goldenrod can be used for health benefits, it's crucial to tell them apart from toxic lookalikes like ragwort. If you're not sure, check a local field guide. Goldenrod leaves are alternately arranged, often toothed, and the plant's shape varies by species. As the plant grows, the base leaves are longer, with the top leaves getting shorter, all with three clear veins. The stems stay single until it's flower time, with yellow florets making up the heads, which might have a few or many florets. Flower heads are typically small, but some types have larger ones. Goldenrods range from 2 to 5 feet tall, with some spreading fast and others growing in expanding clumps.

Uses

1. Goldenrod's astringent and antiseptic qualities make it great for urinary and bladder infections, helping the kidneys and preventing stones. It's a diuretic, so it's better for long-term issues than acute ones.

2. It boosts digestion and soothes inflammation that leads to diarrhea, tackling both symptoms and causes with its anti-inflammatory and anti-microbial powers.

3. Loaded with rutin, an antioxidant, goldenrod supports the heart and blood vessels, enhancing circulation and fortifying capillaries. Those needing these benefits often drink Goldenrod Tea, unless they have blood pressure concerns.

4. Its antifungal properties combat yeast infections like Candida. You can drink the tea or use the decoction, and apply powdered goldenrod for external infections. For oral thrush, a goldenrod gargle can be effective.

5. Goldenrod is perfect for healing skin wounds, burns, and irritations, thanks to its anti-inflammatory, antibacterial, and antifungal actions. It speeds up healing and eases discomfort. Goldenrod can be applied topically to wounds as a poultice, wash, or occasionally even as dried powdered leaves. It's been dubbed "woundwort" for its bleeding-stopping abilities, especially in powdered form. Goldenrod can also be made into ointments for burns.

6. For seasonal allergies and colds, Goldenrod Tincture is a solid pick. It eases watery eyes, runny noses, and sneezing. With antiseptic and expectorant qualities, plus natural antihistamines like quercetin and rutin, it also soothes sore throats. Drinking it as tea works too, and for throat relief, mixing it with sage is a good bet.

Preparation:

1. Goldenrod Tea:

- Simple Preparation: Steep dried goldenrod flowers or leaves in hot water to make a tea.
- Usage: Goldenrod tea is traditionally used to promote urinary tract health, relieve inflammation, and support overall wellness. It has a mildly astringent and slightly bitter taste.

2. Goldenrod Tincture:

- Alcohol Extraction: Goldenrod flowers or leaves can be soaked in alcohol to create a tincture.
- Usage: Goldenrod tincture is a concentrated form of the herb that can be taken orally by adding a few drops to water or juice. It is believed to have similar therapeutic effects as the tea but in a more concentrated form.

Safety and Considerations:

Allergic Reactions: Some individuals may be allergic to goldenrod or other plants in the Asteraceae family, such as ragweed, daisies, and marigolds. Use caution if you have known allergies to these plants.

Pregnancy and Breastfeeding: Goldenrod is not recommended for use during pregnancy or breastfeeding due to limited safety data. It may stimulate uterine contractions and cause miscarriage in pregnant women.

Medication Interactions: Goldenrod may interact with certain medications, including diuretics, anticoagulants, and medications metabolized by the liver. Consult with a healthcare provider before using goldenrod supplements or extracts if you are taking medication.

Corydalis, Corydalis yanhusuo

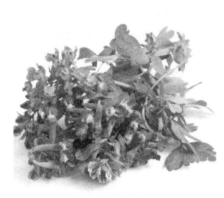

Composition:

- Primary Components: Corydalis contains various alkaloids, including dehydrocorybulbine (DHCB) and tetrahydropalmatine (THP), which are believed to have analgesic, anti-inflammatory, and neuroprotective effects.
- Nutritional Content: Corydalis is not typically consumed for its nutritional content but may contain trace amounts of vitamins, minerals, and other phytochemicals.

Corydalis has been a staple in Chinese medicine since at least the 8th century, used for its ability to stimulate blood flow and ease a wide array of painful ailments. It's especially favored for easing menstrual cramps and pain in the chest and abdomen. Studies in China have backed up its traditional uses, showing that it contains potent alkaloids that give it pain-relieving powers. This plant, native to places like Siberia, northern China, and Japan, is often grown in China's eastern and northeastern regions. It's planted either in early spring or fall, with the rhizome being harvested in late spring or early summer as the plant's above-ground parts start to die back.

Uses

1. It's primarily used to combat pain and is a common component in Chinese herbal remedies for pain relief, typically mixed with other herbs.

2. If you're dealing with period pain, corydalis could be a natural option worth considering, and it pairs nicely with cramp bark.

3. Corydalis is also turned to for various kinds of abdominal pain, from the lower abdomen issues like appendicitis to upper abdomen troubles like peptic ulcers.

4. In the realm of Chinese medicine and other herbal practices, pain is often seen as a result of blocked blood flow. Since corydalis is believed to boost blood circulation, it's particularly helpful for pain linked to injuries.

Preparation:

1. Corydalis Tincture:

- Alcohol Extraction: The tubers of Corydalis yanhusuo can be soaked in alcohol to create a tincture.
- Usage: Corydalis tincture is a concentrated form of the herb that can be taken orally by adding a few drops to water or juice. It is commonly used for its analgesic properties and may help alleviate various types of pain.

2. Corydalis Powder:

- Powdered Form: Dried Corydalis tubers can be ground into a powder.
- Usage: Corydalis powder can be encapsulated for convenient oral consumption or mixed with water or other liquids. It is often used as a natural remedy for pain relief.

Safety and Considerations:

Dosage Considerations: Corydalis should be used at appropriate dosages and under the guidance of a qualified healthcare provider. Excessive consumption may cause adverse effects or interactions with medications.

Pregnancy and Breastfeeding: Corydalis is not recommended for use during pregnancy or breastfeeding due to limited safety data. It may affect hormone levels and could potentially harm the developing fetus or nursing infant.

Medication Interactions: Corydalis may interact with certain medications, including sedatives, antidepressants, and blood thinners. Consult with a healthcare provider before using Corydalis supplements or extracts if you are taking medication.

Henbane, Hyoscyamus niger

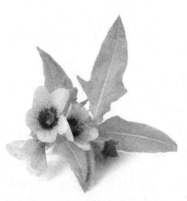

Composition:

- **Primary Components:** Henbane contains various alkaloids, including hyoscyamine, scopolamine, and atropine, which are potent anticholinergic substances. These alkaloids are responsible for the plant's psychoactive and toxic effects.
- **Toxicity:** All parts of the Henbane plant, especially the leaves and seeds, are highly toxic and can cause severe poisoning if ingested. The alkaloids present in Henbane can cause hallucinations, delirium, convulsions, respiratory depression, and death.

Henbane is known for its toxicity, so handle it carefully. This plant, originally from Europe, has been grown in North America for quite some time. It's a real looker despite its stinky reputation and belongs to the Nightshade family. The Hyoscyamus niger plant can reach between one to three feet in height. When henbane matures, it sports bushy, hairy stems that stand tall and branch out. It's a plant that completes its life cycle over two years, and it's the second year's growth that's harvested for medicinal use. Henbane's leaves are a bit stinky, with a grayish or yellowish-green hue and distinctive white veins. They fan out in a rosette pattern, are pretty large and toothed, and can grow up to 6 inches wide and 8 inches long. The flowers, which bloom from June to September, are funnel-shaped, brownish-yellow with dark purple veins, and can be as wide as 2 inches. They grow in a spiky pattern along the upper leaves, with the younger blooms at the tip. The urn-shaped fruit is about an inch big and crammed with loads of tiny black seeds. Henbane's roots are pale and have a thick, branched main taproot. It's not a fan of soggy soil and prefers hanging out in pastures or along fences and roadsides.

Uses

1. Henbane can soothe an irritated bladder and ease the discomfort of cystitis. It acts as a gentle diuretic, sedative, and muscle relaxant. Its sedative effects are similar to those of belladonna but less intense. Exercise extreme caution if you decide to use it, or better yet, opt for a safer alternative, as misuse could be deadly.

2. For those dealing with the discomfort of external hemorrhoids, applying a poultice made from mashed henbane leaves might help bring down the swelling and pain.

3. If you're battling pain from conditions like gout, neuralgia, or arthritis, a fresh henbane leaf poultice could be your go-to remedy. Just crush the leaves and apply them right where it hurts.

Preparation:

- Avoidance: Due to its extreme toxicity, Henbane should not be prepared or used for any purpose, including medicinal or recreational use. Ingesting even small amounts of Henbane can lead to severe poisoning and potentially fatal consequences.

Safety and Considerations:

Extreme Toxicity: Henbane is one of the most toxic plants found in nature. It should never be ingested, handled without gloves, or used for any purpose, including ornamental planting.

Legal Status: Due to its toxicity and potential for misuse, Henbane is regulated in many countries, and its cultivation, sale, or possession may be restricted or prohibited.

Medical Attention: If accidental ingestion or exposure to Henbane occurs, it is essential to seek immediate medical attention. Treatment may involve supportive care, administration of activated charcoal, and symptomatic management of poisoning.

Hawthorn, Crataegus oxyacantha & C. monogyna

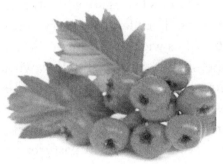

Composition:

• **Primary Components:** Hawthorn contains various bioactive compounds, including flavonoids (such as vitexin, hyperoside, and quercetin), oligomeric procyanidins, triterpenoid acids, and phenolic acids. These compounds are believed to contribute to Hawthorn's cardiovascular benefits.

• **Nutritional Content:** Hawthorn is not typically consumed for its nutritional content but may contain small amounts of vitamins, minerals, and antioxidants.

Hawthorn is highly regarded for its healing properties. Back in the medieval times, it was cherished as a beacon of hope and used to treat various health issues. These days, its primary application is in managing heart and blood vessel conditions, especially angina. Herbalists in the West often describe it as a 'heart tonic,' given its ability to boost blood flow to the heart muscle and help maintain a regular heartbeat. Recent studies have supported these traditional uses. You'll find hawthorn trees dotting the countryside, along roads, and in fields all over the British Isles and other temperate zones in the northern hemisphere. Although you can grow them from seeds, they take a year and a half to sprout, so most people grow them from cuttings instead. The best time to collect the flowers is in the late spring, while the berries are usually picked from late summer to early fall.

Uses

1. In the past, particularly in Europe, hawthorn was a go-to remedy for kidney and bladder stones, and it was also used to promote urination. Herbal manuals from the 16th and 18th centuries, including those by Gerard, Culpeper, and K'Eogh, all mention these applications. However, its modern-day reputation for addressing heart and circulation issues began with an Irish doctor who, in the late 1800s, found it effective for such conditions.

2. Nowadays, hawthorn is commonly recommended for heart-related conditions like angina and coronary artery disease. It's known to enhance heart function and is helpful for mild cases of congestive heart failure and arrhythmias. Hawthorn doesn't produce instant results; it gently works in harmony with the body's natural rhythms, so improvements take some time.

3. Think of hawthorn as a blood pressure regulator. It's particularly good at bringing down high blood pressure, but it also has a knack for bolstering low blood pressure when that's an issue.

4. When paired with ginkgo (Ginkgo biloba), hawthorn can help sharpen a fading memory. This combo is believed to boost blood flow to the brain, which in turn, supplies it with more oxygen, potentially enhancing cognitive function.

Preparation:

1. Hawthorn Tea:

- Simple Preparation: Steep dried Hawthorn berries, leaves, or flowers in hot water to make a tea.
- Usage: Hawthorn tea is traditionally used to support heart health, improve circulation, and promote overall cardiovascular well-being. It tastes tangy and somewhat sweet.

2. Hawthorn Tincture:

- Alcohol Extraction: Hawthorn berries, leaves, or flowers can be soaked in alcohol to create a tincture.
- Usage: Hawthorn tincture is a concentrated form of the herb that can be taken orally by adding a few drops to water or juice. It is commonly used for its cardiovascular benefits and may help regulate blood pressure and cholesterol levels.

Safety and Considerations:

Generally Safe: Hawthorn is considered safe for most people when used appropriately. However, individuals with pre-existing medical conditions, particularly cardiovascular disorders, should consult with a healthcare provider before using Hawthorn supplements.
Medication Interactions: Hawthorn may interact with certain medications, including beta-blockers, calcium channel blockers, digoxin, and anticoagulants. Consult with a healthcare provider before using Hawthorn supplements or extracts if you are taking medication.

4

Conclusion

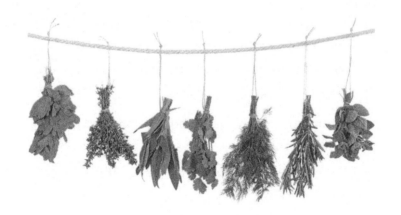

Embracing the Healing Power of Plants

In a realm where man-made drugs tend to rule the healthcare scene, the enchanting promise of plant-based cures presents an intriguing option. For ages, in various cultures and societies, people have turned to Mother Nature for comfort and healing, tapping into the vast array of therapeutic traits hidden within the essence of plants—be it herbs, roots, blossoms, or leaves. This age-old practice of using plants for healing, which stretches from ancient times to today, is a powerful symbol of the lasting bond between us and the earth. From the time-honored knowledge of traditional healers to the detailed studies by today's researchers, the effectiveness of plant remedies has stood the test of time, bringing solace and recovery to many in search of relief from their health woes. Plants, with their complex biochemical makeup and beneficial compounds, offer a way of healing that's in tune with our bodies' natural repair mechanisms. Unlike man-made medicines that usually go after particular symptoms, plant-based treatments work in sync with our systems, tackling the underlying causes of sickness and fostering overall health.

Take, for example, the simple act of sipping a warm mug of chamomile tea to calm jangled nerves, applying aloe vera to soothe a sunburn, or breathing in the scent of eucalyptus to clear stuffy airways—the range and success of plant remedies are truly limitless. Each plant is a treasure trove of healing possibilities, just waiting to be discovered and put to good use for our health. But it's more than just their healing abilities; connecting with the power of plants deepens our bond with the environment. As we interact with these green allies, we're on a path of exploration and reconnection, delving into the complex web of life that links us to the planet and its other inhabitants. From the vivid colors of a blooming garden to the rich aroma of the forest ground, the natural world invites us to dive into its splendor and abundance, urging us to grasp a more profound sense of how all life is interwoven.

In short, turning to plants for healing isn't just about seeking cures; it's about adopting a lifestyle of balance, sustainability, and respect for nature. Through our partnership with the plant kingdom, we gain not only wellness but also a renewed appreciation for the knowledge and marvels at the core of herbal medicine.

Empowering Yourself with Herbal Wisdom:

Where it often feels like health advice is handed down from on high, learning about herbs can be a breath of fresh air. It gives us the power to take care of ourselves. Knowing about herbs isn't just about memorizing their uses; it's about integrating them into our daily routine to stay healthy and happy. Diving into the world of herbalism equips us with powerful tools for steering our own health. Whether we're nurturing a small garden of healing herbs or whipping up natural remedies in our kitchen, we're taking back control. We're not just on the receiving end of health care anymore; we're actively shaping our future with the help of nature's gentle gifts.

But the benefits of herbs aren't limited to just our physical health; they also support our mental, emotional, and spiritual well-being. Simple acts like enjoying a calming cup of herbal tea or basking in the scents of essential oils can unlock the deep healing powers of plants, caring for our whole selves. Herbalism is more than a means to an end—it's a full-circle way of life that brings us into balance with ourselves and the environment. In the end, getting to know herbs is about more than just gathering facts; it's about adopting a mindset of independence, exploration, and self-care. It's about recognizing our body's natural intelligence and nature's limitless capacity for healing, and developing a meaningful, reciprocal bond with the plants that have been our companions since the dawn of time. By doing this, we're not just treating ourselves—we're also paying tribute to the age-old knowledge that beats at the heart of the natural world.

Resources for Further Study and Exploration:

If you're keen to dive into the rich world of herbal medicine, there's a treasure trove of resources waiting for you, ripe with opportunities for further study and discovery. You've got books that range from time-honored texts to the latest research, all brimming with herbal wisdom. These books are treasure chests, filled with age-old practices and cutting-edge science, offering a solid foundation in both the theory and application of herbal medicine. They're perfect for anyone looking to boost their knowledge and sharpen their herbalism skills. But it's not just about flipping through pages. The online world is bustling with ways to learn and get involved. You can join interactive online classes and workshops from the comfort of your living room, guided by seasoned herbal experts. These programs tackle everything from the nitty-gritty of herbs to crafting your own remedies and understanding herbal therapy. With platforms like the Herbal Academy or the Chestnut School of Herbal Medicine, there's something for everyone, no matter if you're just starting out or you're an old hand at this.

Don't forget about the power of community, either. Getting one-on-one advice from professional herbalists can give you custom tips that fit just right for your personal situation. And then there are the local herb walks and events where you can get your hands dirty and meet others who share your passion. It's about building friendships and learning from each other, whether you're at a local meet-up or part of an online group. By tapping into these varied resources, you can really deepen your grasp of herbalism, polish your practice, and set off on an exciting, lifelong adventure in the world of plant-based healing. Whether it's through the wisdom in books, the interactivity of digital courses, or the warmth of community gatherings, the inviting universe of herbal medicine is ready for you to jump in and experience the magic of nature and the healing prowess of plants.

Made in the USA
Monee, IL
13 August 2024

63789717R10077